This publication is intended to provide educational information for the reader on the covered subjects. It is not intended to take the place of personalized medical counseling, diagnosis, and treatment from a trained healthcare professional.

ISBN 978-1-998740-10-9 (Paperback)
ISBN 978-1-998740-09-3 (eBook)

Printed and bound in USA
Published by Loons Press

I0096740

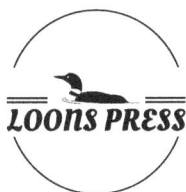

LOONS PRESS

Table Of Contents

Chapter 1   7

Understanding Arrhythmia   7

    What is Arrhythmia?   7

    Types of Arrhythmia   10

    Symptoms and Risks   12

Chapter 2   17

The Heart and Its Function   17

    Anatomy of the Heart   17

    How the Heart Beats   20

    The Role of Electrical Signals   24

Chapter 3   28

Lifestyle Factors   28

    Diet and Nutrition   28

    Physical Activity   31

    Weight Management   34

Chapter 4   38

Managing Stress 38

    Understanding Stress and the Heart 38

    Techniques for Reducing Stress 41

    The Impact of Sleep on Heart Health 44

Chapter 5 48

Avoiding Stimulants 48

    Caffeine and Its Effects 48

    Alcohol Consumption 51

    Smoking and Nicotine 54

Chapter 6 58

Medical Conditions 58

    Hypertension 58

    Diabetes 61

    Thyroid Disorders 64

Chapter 7 69

Medications and Supplements 69

    Common Medications That Affect Heart Rhythm 69

    Heart-Healthy Supplements 72

Consultation   with   Healthcare
Providers   75

Chapter 8   **79**

Monitoring Your Heart Health   **79**

Importance of Regular Check-Ups   79

Home Monitoring Devices   82

Recognizing Warning Signs   85

Chapter 9   **89**

When to Seek Medical Attention   **89**

Understanding Emergency Symptoms   89

Preparing for Doctor Visits   92

Treatment Options for Arrhythmia   95

Chapter 10   **99**

Building a Support System   **99**

The Role of Family and Friends   99

Support Groups and Resources   102

Mental Health Support   105

Chapter 11   **110**

Creating a Personalized Plan   **110**

Assessing Your Risk Factors   110

Setting Goals for a Healthier Heart   113

Regularly Updating Your Plan   116

Chapter 12   **120**

Staying Informed   **120**

Reliable Sources of Information   120

The Importance of Continuing
Education   123

Engaging with Healthcare
Professionals   127

Author Notes & Acknowledgments   **130**

Author Bio   **132**

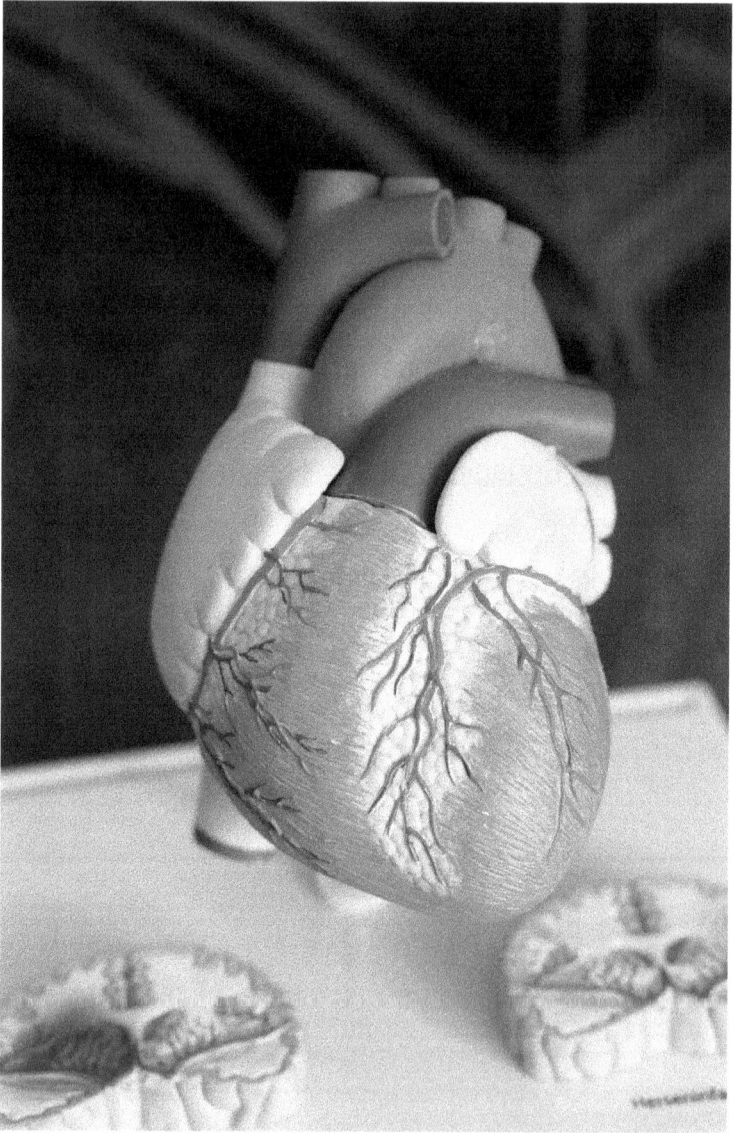

Chapter 1

Understanding Arrhythmia

What is Arrhythmia?

Arrhythmia refers to an irregular heartbeat, which can manifest as a heart that beats too quickly, too slowly, or with an irregular rhythm. This condition can arise from various factors, including heart disease, changes in the heart's structure, or electrical signaling issues within the heart.

While some arrhythmias are benign and may not require treatment, others can lead to serious complications such as stroke, heart failure, or sudden cardiac arrest. Understanding arrhythmia is crucial for those looking to reduce their risk and maintain a healthy heart.

The heart's electrical system governs its rhythm, ensuring that it beats in a coordinated and efficient manner. When this system is disrupted, it can lead to arrhythmias. The heart consists of several components, including the atria and ventricles, which work together to pump blood throughout the body.

If the electrical signals that coordinate these actions become erratic, the heart may not function properly. Common types of arrhythmias include atrial fibrillation, bradycardia, and ventricular tachycardia, each with distinct characteristics and potential health implications.

Risk factors for developing arrhythmia can include lifestyle choices, underlying health conditions, and genetic predispositions. Factors such as excessive alcohol consumption, smoking, high blood pressure, and obesity can increase the likelihood of developing an irregular heartbeat. Additionally, conditions like diabetes, sleep apnea, and thyroid disorders can also contribute. Being aware of these risk factors is essential for individuals aiming to take proactive steps toward heart health and arrhythmia prevention.

Symptoms of arrhythmia can vary significantly from person to person. Some individuals may experience palpitations, dizziness, or light-headedness, while others may have no symptoms at all. In more severe cases, arrhythmias can lead to fainting or chest pain. Recognizing these symptoms is vital, as early intervention can prevent more serious complications. Individuals who suspect they may have an arrhythmia should consult a healthcare professional for proper diagnosis and management.

Preventing arrhythmia involves a multifaceted approach that includes lifestyle modifications and regular health check-ups. Maintaining a balanced diet, engaging in regular physical activity, managing stress, and avoiding tobacco and excessive alcohol are key strategies for promoting heart health.

Furthermore, routine screenings for blood pressure, cholesterol levels, and other cardiovascular risk factors can help identify potential issues early on. By adopting these practices, individuals can significantly reduce their risk of arrhythmia and enhance their overall cardiovascular health.

Types of Arrhythmia

Arrhythmia refers to irregular heartbeats that can manifest in various forms, each with distinct characteristics and implications. Understanding the different types of arrhythmias is crucial for anyone looking to reduce their risk and maintain a healthy heart. The most common types include atrial fibrillation, atrial flutter, and ventricular tachycardia. Each type can affect the heart's ability to pump blood effectively, leading to potential complications if left untreated.

Atrial fibrillation (AFib) is one of the most prevalent forms of arrhythmia. It occurs when the heart's upper chambers, or atria, experience chaotic electrical signals, resulting in a rapid and irregular heartbeat. AFib can lead to symptoms such as palpitations, fatigue, and shortness of breath.

More importantly, it increases the risk of stroke and other heart-related complications, making awareness and management vital for those at risk. Regular check-ups and monitoring can help detect AFib early and allow for timely intervention.

Atrial flutter is similar to AFib but features a more organized electrical circuit in the atria, leading to a rapid but more regular heartbeat. This type of arrhythmia can also contribute to the risk of stroke and heart failure.

Recognizing the symptoms, which may include lightheadedness and chest discomfort, is essential for individuals who may be predisposed to this condition. Lifestyle modifications, like reducing alcohol intake and managing stress, can play a significant role in mitigating the risk of developing atrial flutter.

Ventricular tachycardia (VT) represents a more serious form of arrhythmia that originates in the heart's lower chambers, or ventricles. VT can lead to a significant decrease in cardiac output and may result in fainting or even sudden cardiac arrest in severe cases.

Individuals with underlying heart conditions, such as coronary artery disease or cardiomyopathy, are particularly vulnerable. Prompt medical attention is critical in cases of VT, and understanding one's risk factors can help in preventive strategies.

Other types of arrhythmias include premature atrial contractions (PACs) and premature ventricular contractions (PVCs), which are often benign but can be indicative of underlying heart issues. While occasional PACs and PVCs may not pose a significant risk, frequent occurrences should be evaluated by a healthcare professional.

Monitoring heart health through regular check-ups, maintaining a balanced diet, and engaging in physical activity can significantly reduce the likelihood of these arrhythmias developing into more severe conditions. By understanding the various types of arrhythmias, individuals can take proactive steps to safeguard their heart health and reduce their risk effectively.

Symptoms and Risks

Arrhythmia, a condition characterized by irregular heartbeats, can manifest in various symptoms that may vary in severity and frequency. Common symptoms include palpitations, which are often felt as a fluttering or racing sensation in the chest.

Individuals may also experience dizziness or lightheadedness, especially during physical activity. In some cases, arrhythmia can lead to shortness of breath or fatigue, making everyday tasks feel more strenuous. Recognizing these symptoms early can be crucial in seeking timely medical intervention and managing overall heart health.

The risks associated with arrhythmia extend beyond mere discomfort. Certain types of arrhythmia can lead to serious complications, including stroke, heart failure, or sudden cardiac arrest.

For instance, atrial fibrillation, the most common form of arrhythmia, increases the risk of blood clots forming in the heart. These clots can then travel to the brain, resulting in a stroke. Understanding these potential consequences highlights the importance of addressing arrhythmia symptoms promptly and taking proactive measures to mitigate associated risks.

Several factors can heighten the risk of developing arrhythmia. Age is a significant contributor, as the risk increases with advancing years. Additionally, underlying health conditions such as hypertension, diabetes, and coronary artery disease can create a more favorable environment for arrhythmias to develop.

Lifestyle choices, including excessive alcohol consumption, smoking, and sedentary behavior, also play a critical role in increasing risk. Identifying and modifying these risk factors is essential for anyone looking to reduce their chances of experiencing arrhythmia.

Stress is another crucial element that can exacerbate arrhythmias. Chronic stress can lead to an increase in heart rate and blood pressure, putting additional strain on the cardiovascular system. Moreover, stress often prompts individuals to engage in unhealthy coping mechanisms, such as overeating or substance use, further jeopardizing heart health. Developing effective stress management techniques, such as mindfulness, exercise, or counseling, is an important strategy in the prevention of arrhythmias.

To effectively reduce the risk of arrhythmia, individuals should engage in regular health screenings and maintain open communication with healthcare providers. A thorough understanding of personal health history and risk factors can guide preventative measures and lifestyle adjustments.

Emphasizing heart-healthy habits, such as a balanced diet, regular physical activity, and adequate sleep, can contribute significantly to reducing the likelihood of arrhythmia. By being informed about the symptoms and risks, individuals can empower themselves to take proactive steps toward a healthier heart.

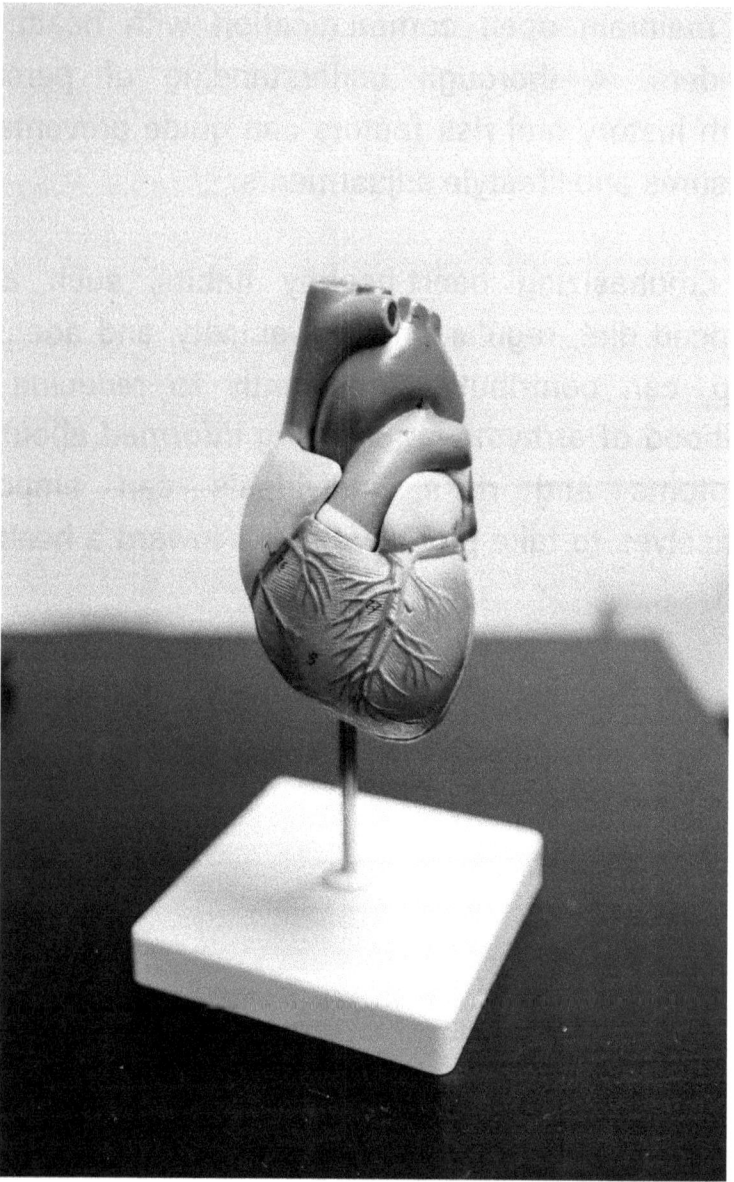

Chapter 2

The Heart and Its Function

Anatomy of the Heart

The heart is a remarkable organ, meticulously designed to pump blood throughout the body, supplying oxygen and nutrients while removing waste products. Its anatomy consists of four chambers: the right atrium, right ventricle, left atrium, and left ventricle. The right atrium receives deoxygenated blood from the body, which then moves to the right ventricle, where it is pumped to the lungs for oxygenation.

Meanwhile, the left atrium collects oxygen-rich blood from the lungs, passing it to the left ventricle, which then pumps it out to the rest of the body. Understanding this structure is crucial for recognizing how arrhythmias can disrupt normal heart function.

The heart's chambers are separated by valves that ensure unidirectional blood flow, preventing backflow. The tricuspid valve sits between the right atrium and right ventricle, while the pulmonary valve is located between the right ventricle and the pulmonary artery.

The mitral valve separates the left atrium from the left ventricle, and the aortic valve is positioned between the left ventricle and the aorta. These valves open and close in response to pressure changes within the heart, and any dysfunction in this system can lead to arrhythmias, characterized by irregular heartbeats.

Central to the heart's function is the electrical conduction system, which coordinates the heartbeat. The sinoatrial (SA) node, located in the right atrium, acts as the natural pacemaker, generating electrical impulses that initiate each heartbeat. These impulses travel through the atria, causing them to contract and push blood into the ventricles. The impulses then reach the atrioventricular (AV) node, which serves as a gatekeeper, delaying the signal before it moves to the ventricles.

This carefully timed process ensures that the chambers contract in a synchronized manner. Disruption in this electrical pathway can lead to various types of arrhythmias.

Cardiac muscle, or myocardium, makes up the heart's walls and is responsible for contraction. The myocardium is thicker in the ventricles than in the atria, reflecting the greater force required to pump blood to the lungs and the rest of the body. The health of the myocardium is vital for maintaining normal rhythm; conditions such as hypertrophy, where the heart muscle thickens, can lead to arrhythmias.

Additionally, the heart is surrounded by a protective sac called the pericardium, which contains fluid that reduces friction during heartbeats. Understanding these structures is essential for identifying potential risks and implementing preventive strategies against arrhythmias.

The coronary arteries supply blood to the heart muscle itself, and any blockage or narrowing of these arteries can result in ischemia, leading to arrhythmias. Maintaining healthy coronary arteries through lifestyle choices such as a balanced diet, regular exercise, and avoiding smoking is crucial for heart health.

Furthermore, factors such as high blood pressure, diabetes, and obesity can negatively impact heart structure and function, increasing the risk of arrhythmias. By understanding the anatomy of the heart and the interconnectedness of its components, individuals can take proactive steps to reduce their risk of arrhythmia and promote overall cardiovascular health.

How the Heart Beats

The heart is a remarkable organ that functions as the body's engine, tirelessly pumping blood to supply oxygen and nutrients to tissues while removing waste products. At its core, the heart's ability to beat is governed by a complex electrical system.

This system is initiated by the sinoatrial (SA) node, often referred to as the natural pacemaker. The SA node generates electrical impulses that spread throughout the heart muscle, coordinating its contractions. This intricate process ensures the heart beats rhythmically, allowing for efficient circulation. Understanding how the heart beats is crucial for individuals looking to reduce their risk of arrhythmia.

When the electrical impulses from the SA node reach the atria, they trigger contraction, pushing blood into the ventricles. This process is followed by the impulses traveling to the atrioventricular (AV) node, which acts as a gatekeeper. The AV node briefly delays the signals, allowing the ventricles to fill with blood before contracting.

This sequence of contraction and relaxation creates the heartbeat, typically measured in beats per minute (BPM). A healthy resting heart rate for adults generally ranges from 60 to 100 BPM. Deviations from this range, whether too fast (tachycardia) or too slow (bradycardia), can indicate potential arrhythmias.

Several factors can influence the heart's electrical system and its ability to maintain a regular rhythm. Stress, caffeine, alcohol, and certain medications can all disrupt the heart's normal functioning. Additionally, underlying health conditions such as high blood pressure, diabetes, and heart disease can contribute to arrhythmia risk.

For those seeking to reduce their risk, it is essential to identify and manage these factors proactively. Lifestyle changes, including regular exercise, a balanced diet, and stress management techniques, can significantly improve heart health and reduce the likelihood of arrhythmias.

Regular monitoring of heart health is also a vital component of arrhythmia prevention. Individuals should be aware of their heart rate and rhythm, especially if they experience symptoms such as palpitations, dizziness, or shortness of breath.

Routine check-ups with a healthcare provider can help identify potential issues early on. Advanced diagnostic tools, such as electrocardiograms (ECGs) or Holter monitors, can provide valuable insights into heart function and detect irregularities that may predispose someone to arrhythmias.

In conclusion, understanding how the heart beats is fundamental for anyone interested in reducing their risk of arrhythmia. By recognizing the role of the electrical system, being aware of influencing factors, and actively monitoring heart health, individuals can take meaningful steps toward ensuring a healthier heart.

Implementing lifestyle changes and seeking professional guidance can empower individuals to maintain a stable heart rhythm, significantly lowering the risk of arrhythmias and promoting overall cardiovascular wellness.

The Role of Electrical Signals

The heart's ability to pump blood efficiently relies heavily on electrical signals that coordinate its contractions. These signals originate from specialized cells in the sinoatrial (SA) node, often referred to as the heart's natural pacemaker. The SA node generates electrical impulses that travel through the heart muscle, triggering the atria to contract and push blood into the ventricles.

This process is essential for maintaining a regular heartbeat, and any disruption in these electrical signals can lead to arrhythmias, which are irregular heart rhythms that can result in serious health issues.

In a healthy heart, the electrical signals follow a precise pathway through the heart's conduction system. After the SA node fires, the impulses spread to the atrioventricular (AV) node, which serves as a gatekeeper, allowing the signals to pass into the ventricles at a controlled rate.

From the AV node, the signals travel along the bundle of His and into the Purkinje fibers, ensuring synchronized contraction of the ventricles. This intricate system highlights the importance of electrical signals not only in the initiation of heartbeats but also in the overall efficiency of the cardiovascular system.

Factors such as stress, poor diet, and underlying health conditions can interfere with the normal electrical signaling processes. For instance, high levels of stress hormones can lead to increased heart rate and irregular rhythms.

Additionally, electrolyte imbalances, often caused by dehydration or poor dietary choices, can disrupt the electrical pathways and contribute to arrhythmias. It is crucial for individuals aiming to reduce their risk of arrhythmia to recognize these influences and adopt lifestyle changes that promote heart health.

Maintaining proper hydration and a balanced diet rich in essential nutrients can significantly support the heart's electrical system. Foods high in potassium, magnesium, and calcium play a vital role in maintaining normal heart rhythm and function. Regular physical activity also enhances cardiovascular health by improving blood flow and reducing stress levels. Incorporating heart-healthy exercise into daily routines can help regulate electrical signals and strengthen the heart muscle, ultimately decreasing the risk of arrhythmias.

In summary, understanding the role of electrical signals in heart function is fundamental for anyone looking to reduce their risk of arrhythmia. By prioritizing lifestyle choices that support the heart's electrical system—such as managing stress, eating a balanced diet, and engaging in regular exercise—individuals can promote a healthier heart and reduce the likelihood of developing irregular heart rhythms. Taking proactive steps in these areas not only fosters a robust cardiovascular system but also contributes to overall well-being.

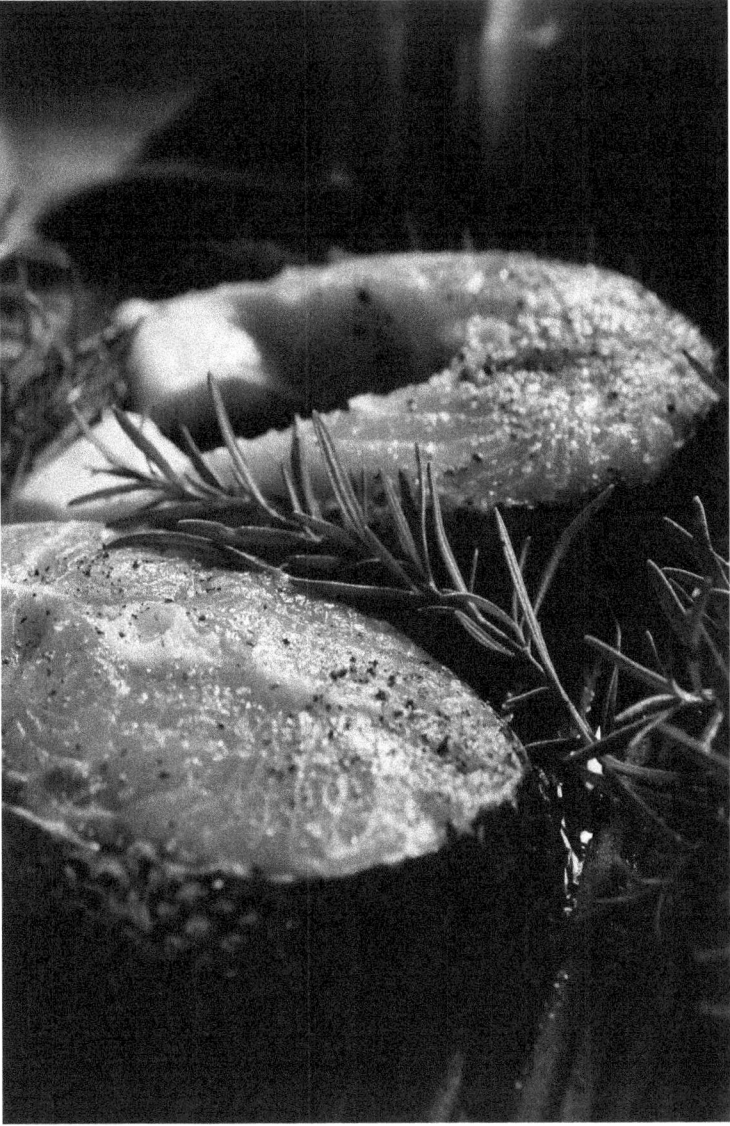

Chapter 3

Lifestyle Factors

Diet and Nutrition

Diet and nutrition play a crucial role in maintaining heart health and can significantly influence the risk of arrhythmia. A well-balanced diet rich in essential nutrients can help manage weight, regulate blood pressure, and improve overall cardiovascular health.

To reduce the risk of arrhythmia, it is essential to focus on foods that promote heart function and limit those that can contribute to heart problems. Adopting a heart-healthy diet is a proactive step individuals can take to protect their heart and maintain a stable rhythm.

Incorporating a variety of fruits and vegetables into daily meals is vital for reducing arrhythmia risk. These foods are rich in vitamins, minerals, and antioxidants, which can help combat oxidative stress and inflammation in the body. Leafy greens, berries, and citrus fruits are particularly beneficial due to their high fiber content and potential to lower blood pressure.

Aim for a colorful plate, as different colors often represent different nutrients that can support heart health. A diet abundant in plant-based foods not only nourishes the body but also helps in maintaining a healthy weight, which is another key factor in reducing arrhythmia risk.

Whole grains should be a staple in a heart-healthy diet. Foods such as brown rice, quinoa, and whole wheat bread provide essential fiber that supports healthy digestion and helps regulate cholesterol levels. This type of fiber can also assist in controlling blood sugar levels, reducing the risk of insulin resistance and diabetes, both of which are risk factors for arrhythmias.

By choosing whole grains over refined options, individuals can ensure they are receiving the maximum nutritional benefits while promoting heart health.

Healthy fats are another critical component of a diet aimed at reducing arrhythmia risk. Incorporating sources of omega-3 fatty acids, such as fatty fish (salmon, mackerel), walnuts, and flaxseeds, can help improve heart rhythm and lower inflammation. These healthy fats support cardiovascular function and have been shown to reduce the incidence of arrhythmias.

It is equally important to minimize the intake of trans fats and saturated fats, often found in processed foods, which can raise cholesterol levels and contribute to heart disease.

Finally, staying hydrated and moderating caffeine and alcohol intake are essential strategies for maintaining a healthy heart. Dehydration can lead to electrolyte imbalances, increasing the likelihood of arrhythmias. Drinking plenty of water throughout the day supports overall health and heart function.

Additionally, while moderate caffeine consumption may not pose a significant risk for everyone, it is wise to monitor its effects on individual heart rhythm. Alcohol, when consumed excessively, can also lead to irregular heartbeats. Thus, moderation is key. By focusing on a balanced diet rich in whole foods, healthy fats, and proper hydration, individuals can take significant steps toward reducing their risk of arrhythmia.

Physical Activity

Physical activity is a crucial component in reducing the risk of arrhythmia and promoting overall heart health. Engaging in regular exercise helps to strengthen the heart muscle, improve circulation, and reduce the likelihood of developing conditions such as high blood pressure and obesity, both of which are risk factors for arrhythmias.

The American Heart Association recommends at least 150 minutes of moderate-intensity aerobic activity or 75 minutes of vigorous activity each week for optimal heart health. Incorporating physical activity into your daily routine can significantly lower your risk of heart-related issues.

Aerobic exercises, such as walking, jogging, swimming, and cycling, are particularly beneficial for cardiovascular health. These activities increase the heart rate and improve blood flow, which can help regulate electrical signals in the heart and prevent arrhythmias.

Additionally, aerobic exercise has been shown to enhance the heart's ability to pump blood efficiently, thereby reducing the strain on the heart. For those who are new to exercise, starting with short, manageable sessions and gradually increasing intensity and duration can make the process more approachable and sustainable.

Strength training also plays a vital role in heart health by building muscle mass and improving metabolic function. A well-rounded exercise routine that includes strength training exercises at least twice a week can help maintain a healthy weight and reduce fat accumulation around the heart, which is a known risk factor for arrhythmias. Resistance exercises, such as weight lifting or bodyweight exercises, can also improve overall body composition and enhance physical endurance, further supporting cardiovascular health.

Flexibility and balance exercises, such as yoga and tai chi, are equally important for heart health and can contribute to reducing arrhythmia risk. These activities promote relaxation and stress reduction, which are essential for maintaining a healthy heart. Chronic stress and anxiety can lead to increased heart rate and blood pressure, potentially triggering arrhythmias.

By incorporating relaxation techniques and gentle movement into your routine, you can create a holistic approach to managing heart health and reducing risk factors.

Before starting any new exercise program, particularly for individuals with existing health conditions or those who have experienced arrhythmias, consulting with a healthcare professional is critical. They can help tailor an exercise plan that is safe and effective based on individual health status. By committing to a consistent physical activity routine, individuals can take proactive steps toward reducing their risk of arrhythmia and fostering a healthier heart for the long term.

Weight Management

Weight management plays a critical role in reducing the risk of arrhythmia, as excess body weight can contribute to various cardiovascular issues. Obesity is linked to an increased risk of developing conditions such as high blood pressure, diabetes, and sleep apnea, all of which can exacerbate heart rhythm disorders.

Maintaining a healthy weight can help alleviate these risk factors and promote overall heart health. By adopting lifestyle changes that focus on weight management, individuals can significantly decrease their likelihood of experiencing arrhythmias.

To achieve effective weight management, it is essential to adopt a balanced diet rich in whole foods. Emphasizing fruits, vegetables, whole grains, lean proteins, and healthy fats can provide the necessary nutrients while promoting satiety. Reducing the intake of processed foods, added sugars, and unhealthy fats is equally important, as these can contribute to weight gain and negatively impact heart health.

Keeping a food diary can also help individuals become more aware of their eating habits and make healthier choices.

In addition to dietary changes, regular physical activity is crucial for weight management and heart health. Engaging in at least 150 minutes of moderate-intensity aerobic exercise each week can help burn calories and improve cardiovascular fitness. Activities such as brisk walking, cycling, swimming, and dancing not only help maintain a healthy weight but also enhance the heart's efficiency.

Incorporating strength training exercises at least two days a week can further support weight loss efforts and build muscle, which increases metabolic rate and aids in weight maintenance.

Behavioral strategies also play an important role in successful weight management. Setting realistic and achievable goals can help individuals stay motivated and focused on their weight loss journey.

It may be beneficial to seek support from healthcare professionals, such as dietitians or personal trainers, who can provide personalized guidance and accountability. Joining support groups or engaging with friends and family on similar health journeys can foster a sense of community, making the process more enjoyable and sustainable.

Finally, it is essential to recognize that weight management is a lifelong commitment rather than a short-term diet. Developing healthy habits that can be maintained over time will lead to lasting results and improved heart health. Regular monitoring of weight and health markers, along with periodic adjustments to diet and exercise routines, can help individuals stay on track. By prioritizing weight management, individuals can significantly reduce their risk of arrhythmias and enhance their overall quality of life.

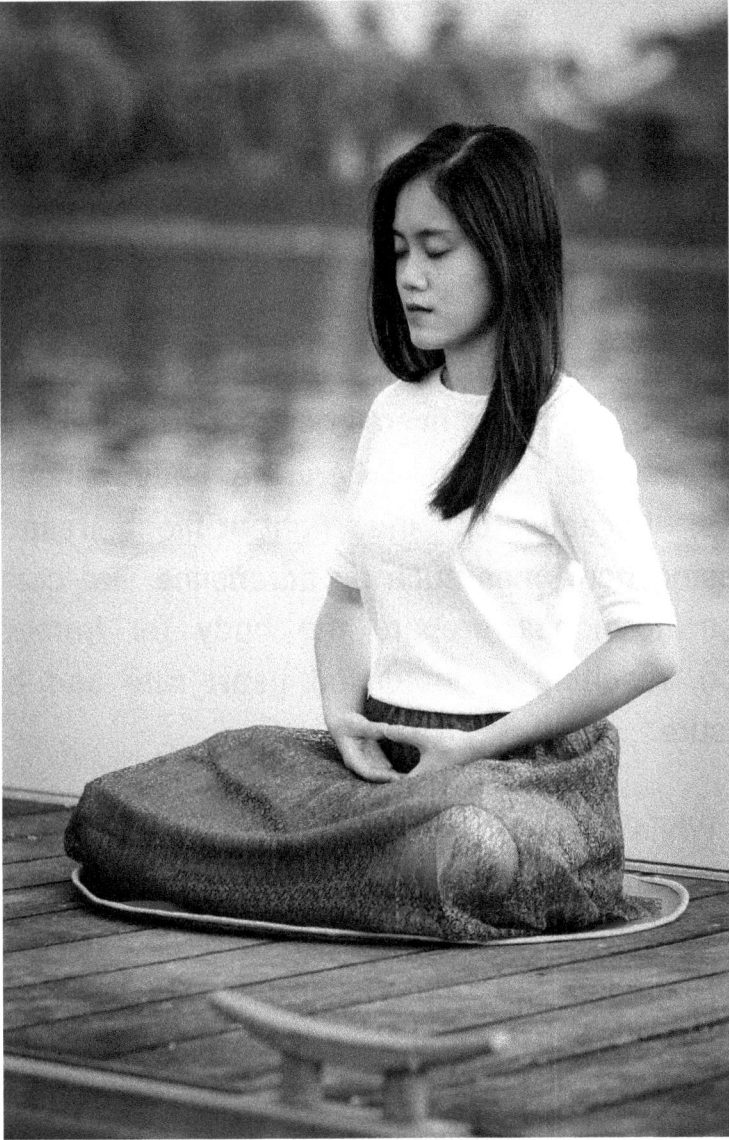

Chapter 4

Managing Stress

Understanding Stress and the Heart

Stress is a common experience that can have significant effects on overall health, particularly on the cardiovascular system. When the body encounters stress, it activates the fight-or-flight response, releasing hormones such as adrenaline and cortisol. These hormones prepare the body for immediate action, resulting in increased heart rate and blood pressure.

While these physiological changes are beneficial in short bursts, chronic stress can lead to long-term cardiovascular issues, including arrhythmias. Understanding the relationship between stress and heart health is essential for anyone looking to reduce their risk of arrhythmia.

One of the primary ways stress impacts the heart is through its effect on the autonomic nervous system, which regulates involuntary bodily functions, including heart rate. Stress can lead to an imbalance in this system, often resulting in increased sympathetic nervous system activity and reduced parasympathetic activity.

This imbalance can contribute to irregular heartbeats, or arrhythmias, making it crucial for individuals to manage their stress levels effectively. Recognizing stress triggers and implementing coping mechanisms is vital for maintaining a healthy heart rhythm.

Chronic stress may also contribute to unhealthy lifestyle choices that further increase the risk of arrhythmia. Individuals experiencing high levels of stress may turn to smoking, excessive alcohol consumption, or poor dietary habits as coping mechanisms. These behaviors can exacerbate heart issues and lead to conditions such as hypertension and obesity, which are known risk factors for arrhythmias.

By addressing stress proactively, individuals can not only improve their emotional well-being but also foster healthier lifestyle choices that support heart health.

Moreover, studies have shown that stress management techniques can have a positive impact on heart health. Practices such as mindfulness meditation, yoga, and regular physical activity have been linked to reduced levels of stress and improved cardiovascular outcomes.

These activities can help lower blood pressure, decrease heart rate, and enhance overall emotional resilience. Incorporating stress reduction strategies into daily life can be a powerful tool for those looking to mitigate their risk of developing arrhythmias.

In conclusion, understanding the connection between stress and heart health is critical for reducing the risk of arrhythmia. By recognizing how stress affects the body and adopting effective stress management techniques, individuals can take proactive steps toward improving their cardiovascular health.

Prioritizing mental well-being, coupled with healthy lifestyle choices, creates a comprehensive approach to heart health that can significantly lower the likelihood of arrhythmias and promote overall wellness.

Techniques for Reducing Stress

Stress is a significant factor that can contribute to the risk of arrhythmia, making it essential for individuals to adopt effective stress-reduction techniques. Various methods can help lower stress levels, ultimately promoting heart health and reducing the likelihood of heart rhythm disorders. Implementing these strategies can lead to a more balanced lifestyle, encouraging both mental and physical well-being.

One widely recommended technique for stress reduction is mindfulness meditation. This practice involves focusing attention on the present moment and cultivating awareness of thoughts and feelings without judgment.

Regularly engaging in mindfulness meditation can help lower blood pressure, reduce anxiety, and improve emotional regulation. For those at risk of arrhythmia, incorporating mindfulness into daily routines may contribute to a calmer state of mind and a healthier heart.

Physical activity is another proven method for alleviating stress. Exercise releases endorphins, which are natural mood lifters, and can help mitigate feelings of anxiety and depression. Activities such as walking, swimming, or yoga not only enhance physical fitness but also promote relaxation.

Engaging in regular exercise can improve heart health, making it an essential component of a comprehensive strategy for reducing the risk of arrhythmia. Aim for at least 150 minutes of moderate-intensity exercise each week to maximize these benefits.

Deep breathing exercises are a simple yet effective way to manage stress. Practicing techniques such as diaphragmatic breathing or the 4-7-8 breathing method can help activate the body's relaxation response, reducing heart rate and promoting a sense of calm. These exercises can be easily incorporated into daily life, whether at home or during moments of heightened stress. By prioritizing deep breathing, individuals can create a powerful tool for managing stress and its impact on heart health.

Finally, fostering social connections can significantly contribute to stress reduction. Building and maintaining relationships with friends, family, and community members provides emotional support and a sense of belonging. Engaging in social activities, sharing experiences, and discussing feelings can alleviate the burden of stress.

For those concerned about arrhythmia, cultivating a strong social network can serve as a buffer against stress, enhancing both mental and cardiovascular health. By integrating these techniques into daily life, individuals can take proactive steps to reduce stress and lower their risk of developing arrhythmia.

The Impact of Sleep on Heart Health

Sleep plays a crucial role in maintaining overall health, and its impact on heart health is particularly significant. Research has shown that insufficient sleep can lead to various cardiovascular issues, including arrhythmias.

When individuals do not get enough restorative sleep, the body experiences heightened levels of stress hormones, such as cortisol, which can contribute to increased heart rate and blood pressure. These physiological changes create an environment conducive to the development of irregular heartbeats, making adequate sleep an essential component of arrhythmia prevention.

Quality sleep is vital for the body's repair processes, including those involving the cardiovascular system. During sleep, the body undergoes various restorative processes, including the regulation of blood pressure and heart rate.

Poor sleep can disrupt these processes, leading to an imbalance in the autonomic nervous system, which controls heart function. This disruption can increase the likelihood of experiencing episodes of arrhythmia. Furthermore, chronic sleep deprivation has been linked to inflammation, which is another factor that can adversely affect heart health.

The relationship between sleep disorders and heart health is also noteworthy. Conditions such as sleep apnea have been shown to significantly increase the risk of developing arrhythmias. Sleep apnea causes repeated interruptions in breathing during sleep, leading to drops in oxygen levels and increased strain on the heart.

This can result in irregular heartbeats and other cardiovascular complications. Addressing sleep disorders not only helps improve sleep quality but also mitigates the risk of arrhythmias and other heart-related issues.

Lifestyle choices play a vital role in ensuring quality sleep and, by extension, heart health. Establishing a consistent sleep schedule, creating a relaxing bedtime routine, and optimizing the sleep environment are essential strategies for enhancing sleep quality. Additionally, reducing the intake of caffeine and alcohol, especially in the hours leading up to bedtime, can further improve sleep. These lifestyle changes can help individuals achieve the restorative sleep necessary for optimal heart function and reduce the risk of arrhythmias.

Incorporating sleep hygiene practices into daily routines can be an effective strategy for reducing the risk of arrhythmia. Individuals should prioritize sleep as an integral part of their overall health strategy, recognizing its profound effects on heart health. By fostering better sleep habits, individuals can not only enhance their quality of life but also take a proactive step in protecting their heart health, ultimately reducing their risk of experiencing arrhythmias.

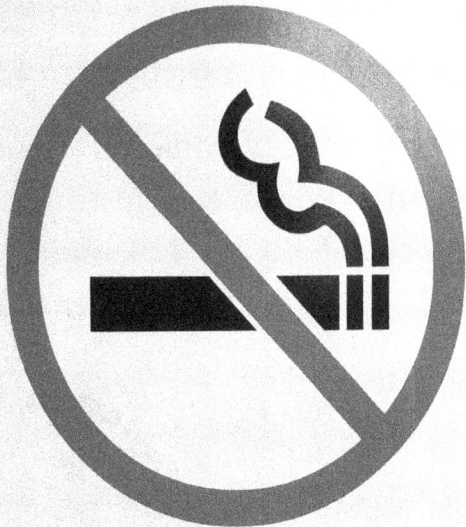

NO
SMOKING

Chapter 5

Avoiding Stimulants

Caffeine and Its Effects

Caffeine is a stimulant commonly found in coffee, tea, chocolate, and various energy drinks. Its primary action is to block adenosine receptors in the brain, which can lead to increased alertness and reduced fatigue.

For many individuals, moderate caffeine consumption is a part of daily life, providing benefits such as improved concentration and enhanced physical performance.

However, it is essential for those looking to reduce their risk of arrhythmia to understand how caffeine can affect heart health, as its stimulatory effects may also have potential drawbacks.

Research has shown that caffeine can increase heart rate and induce palpitations in some individuals, particularly when consumed in high doses. For those with pre-existing heart conditions or a predisposition to arrhythmias, excessive caffeine intake may exacerbate symptoms or trigger irregular heartbeats.

The relationship between caffeine and arrhythmias is complex, as individual tolerance levels and genetic factors play a significant role in how caffeine affects the heart. Thus, understanding personal limits is crucial for anyone concerned about arrhythmia risk.

Moderate caffeine consumption, often defined as 200-400 milligrams per day (about 2-4 cups of brewed coffee), may not pose significant risks for most healthy adults. In fact, some studies suggest that moderate caffeine intake may even be associated with a lower risk of certain cardiovascular diseases. However, individuals with a history of arrhythmias or other heart issues should approach caffeine with caution. Monitoring heart rhythm and symptoms in response to caffeine can help gauge its effects and guide consumption.

For those striving to reduce their risk of arrhythmia, it may be beneficial to consider alternatives to high-caffeine beverages. Herbal teas, decaffeinated coffee, and other non-caffeinated drinks can provide hydration and enjoyment without the potential stimulatory effects of caffeine.

Additionally, adopting a balanced diet rich in fruits, vegetables, whole grains, and omega-3 fatty acids can support overall heart health, potentially mitigating any adverse effects caffeine may have.

Ultimately, the key to managing caffeine consumption lies in moderation and individual awareness. Keeping a food and beverage diary can help track caffeine intake and its correlation with heart rhythm changes. By understanding how caffeine affects their bodies, individuals can make informed choices that align with their heart health goals, thereby reducing their risk of arrhythmia while still enjoying their favorite beverages in moderation.

Alcohol Consumption

Alcohol consumption can have a significant impact on heart health, particularly for individuals concerned about arrhythmia. While moderate alcohol intake may not pose a severe risk for everyone, excessive or even regular consumption can lead to various cardiovascular issues, including the development of arrhythmias. Understanding the relationship between alcohol and heart health is essential for those looking to reduce their risk of arrhythmia.

Research indicates that alcohol can have both direct and indirect effects on the heart. Acute intake of alcohol may trigger arrhythmias in susceptible individuals, leading to conditions like atrial fibrillation. This can occur even after consuming moderate amounts of alcohol in some cases.

The mechanisms behind alcohol-induced arrhythmias are complex, involving alterations in electrolyte balance, changes in heart rate, and increased sympathetic nervous system activity. These factors can disrupt the heart's normal rhythm, making it more susceptible to irregularities.

In addition to the immediate effects of alcohol, chronic consumption poses further risks. Long-term alcohol use can lead to conditions such as cardiomyopathy, which weakens the heart muscle and can precipitate arrhythmias. Those who consume alcohol excessively are also at risk of developing high blood pressure, obesity, and other lifestyle-related factors that contribute to heart disease.

Therefore, individuals aiming to reduce their risk of arrhythmia should be mindful of their drinking habits and consider the cumulative impact of alcohol on their cardiovascular health.

For those who choose to consume alcohol, moderation is key. Health authorities often define moderate drinking as up to one drink per day for women and up to two drinks per day for men. Individuals should also consider their overall health, family history, and any pre-existing heart conditions when evaluating their alcohol consumption.

Keeping a record of drinking habits and being aware of how alcohol affects one's body can help in making informed decisions about beverage choices.

In conclusion, understanding the implications of alcohol consumption is crucial for anyone concerned about arrhythmia. By recognizing the potential risks associated with both moderate and excessive drinking, individuals can take proactive steps to protect their heart health. This includes being mindful of intake levels, seeking alternatives, and engaging in lifestyle changes that promote a healthier heart, ultimately reducing the risk of arrhythmias and enhancing overall well-being.

Smoking and Nicotine

Smoking is a significant risk factor for a variety of cardiovascular diseases, including arrhythmias. The harmful substances found in tobacco products can lead to structural and functional changes in the heart. Smoking increases heart rate and blood pressure, placing extra strain on the cardiovascular system.

This strain can lead to the development of arrhythmias, which are irregular heartbeats that can be both uncomfortable and dangerous. For those looking to reduce their risk of arrhythmia, understanding the impact of smoking and nicotine is crucial.

Nicotine, the primary addictive substance in tobacco, has several effects on the heart. Upon entering the bloodstream, nicotine stimulates the release of adrenaline, which can cause the heart to beat faster and increase blood pressure. This heightened state can provoke episodes of arrhythmia, especially in individuals who may already have underlying heart conditions.

Furthermore, nicotine can also contribute to the hardening of arteries, a condition known as atherosclerosis, which can exacerbate arrhythmic events by diminishing blood flow to the heart.

In addition to nicotine, smoking exposes individuals to a cocktail of harmful chemicals. These include carbon monoxide, formaldehyde, and various heavy metals, all of which can damage heart tissue and disrupt normal electrical signaling in the heart. Research has shown that even secondhand smoke can increase the risk of arrhythmias, making it essential for both smokers and non-smokers to be aware of the dangers associated with tobacco exposure.

Quitting smoking is one of the most effective ways to improve heart health and reduce the likelihood of developing arrhythmias.

The benefits of quitting smoking extend beyond reducing the risk of arrhythmias. Individuals who stop smoking often experience improvements in overall cardiovascular health, including lower blood pressure and improved circulation.

The heart begins to recover from the damaging effects of nicotine and other harmful substances, leading to a more stable heart rhythm. Support programs, counseling, and pharmacological aids can assist those trying to quit, making the transition easier and more sustainable.

In conclusion, addressing smoking and nicotine consumption is a vital strategy for anyone looking to reduce their risk of arrhythmia. The negative impacts of smoking on heart health are well-documented, and the benefits of quitting are profound. By eliminating tobacco use, individuals can significantly lower their chances of developing arrhythmias and enhance their overall heart health. For those committed to making a change, resources are available to support the journey toward a smoke-free life and a healthier heart.

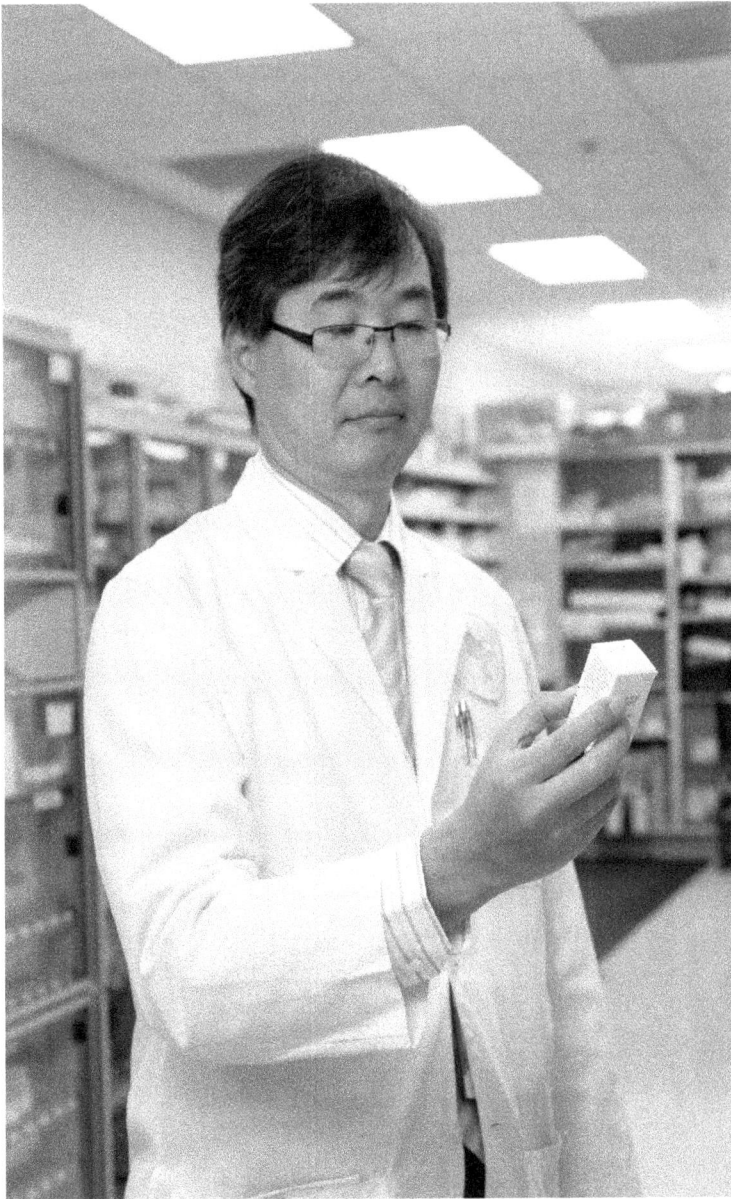

Chapter 6

Medical Conditions

Hypertension

Hypertension, or high blood pressure, is a significant risk factor for various cardiovascular diseases, including arrhythmias. It occurs when the force of the blood against the artery walls is consistently too high, which can lead to damage over time. The heart has to work harder to pump blood, and this increased workload can result in structural changes to the heart, such as left ventricular hypertrophy.

These changes can disrupt the heart's electrical system, leading to abnormal heart rhythms. Understanding hypertension and its management is crucial for anyone looking to reduce their risk of arrhythmia.

There are several causes of hypertension, including lifestyle choices, genetic predispositions, and underlying health conditions. Excessive salt intake, a diet high in saturated fats, lack of physical activity, obesity, and excessive alcohol consumption are common contributors.

Additionally, stress and chronic conditions such as diabetes and kidney disease can elevate blood pressure levels. Recognizing these factors is essential for implementing effective strategies to manage blood pressure and consequently lower the risk of developing arrhythmias.

Preventive measures and lifestyle changes play a pivotal role in managing hypertension. Incorporating a heart-healthy diet, such as the DASH (Dietary Approaches to Stop Hypertension) diet, can significantly lower blood pressure. This diet emphasizes fruits, vegetables, whole grains, and lean proteins while reducing sodium intake.

Regular physical activity is also vital; aiming for at least 150 minutes of moderate exercise per week can help maintain a healthy weight and reduce blood pressure. Furthermore, stress management techniques, such as mindfulness and yoga, can contribute to overall heart health.

In some cases, lifestyle changes may not be sufficient to control hypertension, and medication may be necessary. Various antihypertensive medications are available, including diuretics, ACE inhibitors, beta-blockers, and calcium channel blockers.

Consulting with a healthcare provider is essential for determining the most appropriate treatment plan based on individual circumstances. Regular monitoring of blood pressure is also crucial to ensure that any necessary adjustments to treatment can be made promptly.

Finally, understanding the link between hypertension and arrhythmias underscores the importance of proactive health management. Individuals with high blood pressure should regularly check their blood pressure levels and work closely with doctors develop a comprehensive plan.

By taking charge of their heart health through education, lifestyle modifications, and, if needed, medical intervention, individuals can significantly reduce their risk of arrhythmia and promote a healthier heart.

Diabetes

Diabetes is a chronic condition that significantly influences cardiovascular health. Research indicates that individuals with diabetes, particularly type 2 diabetes, are at a heightened risk for developing arrhythmias. This connection is primarily due to the impact of diabetes on various metabolic processes, leading to complications such as hypertension, obesity, and hyperlipidemia, all of which can contribute to the development of heart rhythm disorders. Understanding this relationship is crucial for individuals seeking to reduce their risk of arrhythmia.

The mechanisms through which diabetes affects heart health are multifaceted. Elevated blood sugar levels can lead to damage of the blood vessels and nerves that control the heart. This damage may result in autonomic dysfunction, which can disrupt the heart's electrical signals and increase the likelihood of arrhythmias.

Additionally, diabetes contributes to the accumulation of fatty deposits in the arteries, promoting atherosclerosis. The narrowing of these arteries can impede blood flow and lead to ischemia, further increasing the risk of arrhythmic events.

Effective management of diabetes is essential not only for controlling blood sugar levels but also for minimizing the risk of arrhythmias. Adopting a balanced diet rich in whole grains, lean proteins, fruits, and vegetables can help manage weight and improve insulin sensitivity.

Regular physical activity plays a vital role in this process, as it can enhance cardiovascular health, lower blood pressure, and reduce body fat. Furthermore, monitoring blood sugar levels consistently allows individuals to make informed decisions about their diet and medication, ultimately leading to better overall health outcomes.

Medication management is another critical component in reducing the risk of arrhythmia for those with diabetes. It is important for individuals to work closely with their healthcare providers to find the most effective treatment regimen.

This may include medications to control blood sugar levels, as well as those that address other cardiovascular risk factors such as hypertension and high cholesterol. Regular check-ups and discussions about medication adjustments can help ensure that individuals maintain optimal heart health.

In conclusion, understanding the link between diabetes and arrhythmia is vital for those looking to protect their heart health. By implementing lifestyle changes, managing blood sugar levels, and adhering to medical advice, individuals can significantly reduce their risk of developing arrhythmias. Proactive measures, including a healthy diet, regular exercise, and proper medication management, are essential strategies for achieving a healthier heart and improving overall well-being.

Thyroid Disorders

Thyroid disorders can significantly impact heart health and are essential to consider when addressing the risk of arrhythmia. The thyroid gland, located in the neck, produces hormones that regulate metabolism, energy levels, and overall bodily functions.

An imbalance in these hormones, whether due to hyperthyroidism (overactive thyroid) or hypothyroidism (underactive thyroid), can lead to various cardiovascular issues, including arrhythmias. Understanding these conditions and their effects on heart function is crucial for anyone looking to maintain a healthy heart.

Hyperthyroidism can lead to an increased heart rate, known as tachycardia, which can trigger arrhythmias. The excess hormones cause the heart to work harder, potentially leading to palpitations, irregular heartbeats, or even more severe complications like atrial fibrillation.

Individuals with hyperthyroidism may notice symptoms such as unexpected weight loss, anxiety, and increased sweating, all of which can contribute to an elevated risk of heart issues. Recognizing these symptoms early and seeking medical advice can help mitigate risks and promote a healthier heart.

Conversely, hypothyroidism can also pose risks to cardiovascular health. An underactive thyroid slows down metabolism and can lead to a slower heart rate, known as bradycardia. This condition can result in poor circulation and increased cholesterol levels, both of which are risk factors for arrhythmia.

Many people with hypothyroidism may experience fatigue, weight gain, and depression, which can further complicate heart health. Regular monitoring of thyroid function is essential for those with symptoms or a family history of thyroid disorders, as timely treatment can help stabilize hormone levels and support heart health.

Managing thyroid disorders often involves medication to regulate hormone levels, which can subsequently reduce the risk of arrhythmias. For hyperthyroidism, treatments may include antithyroid medications, radioactive iodine, or even surgery in severe cases.

For hypothyroidism, thyroid hormone replacement therapy is usually effective. It's vital for individuals undergoing treatment to work closely with their healthcare providers to monitor heart health, adjusting treatments as necessary to ensure optimal functioning of both the thyroid and the heart.

Preventive measures can also play a significant role in reducing the risk of arrhythmias related to thyroid disorders. Maintaining a balanced diet rich in nutrients that support thyroid function, such as iodine, selenium, and zinc, can help regulate hormone levels. Regular exercise, stress management techniques, and routine medical check-ups are equally important in managing both thyroid health and heart health. By being proactive and informed about thyroid disorders, individuals can take meaningful steps to protect their hearts and reduce their risk of arrhythmia.

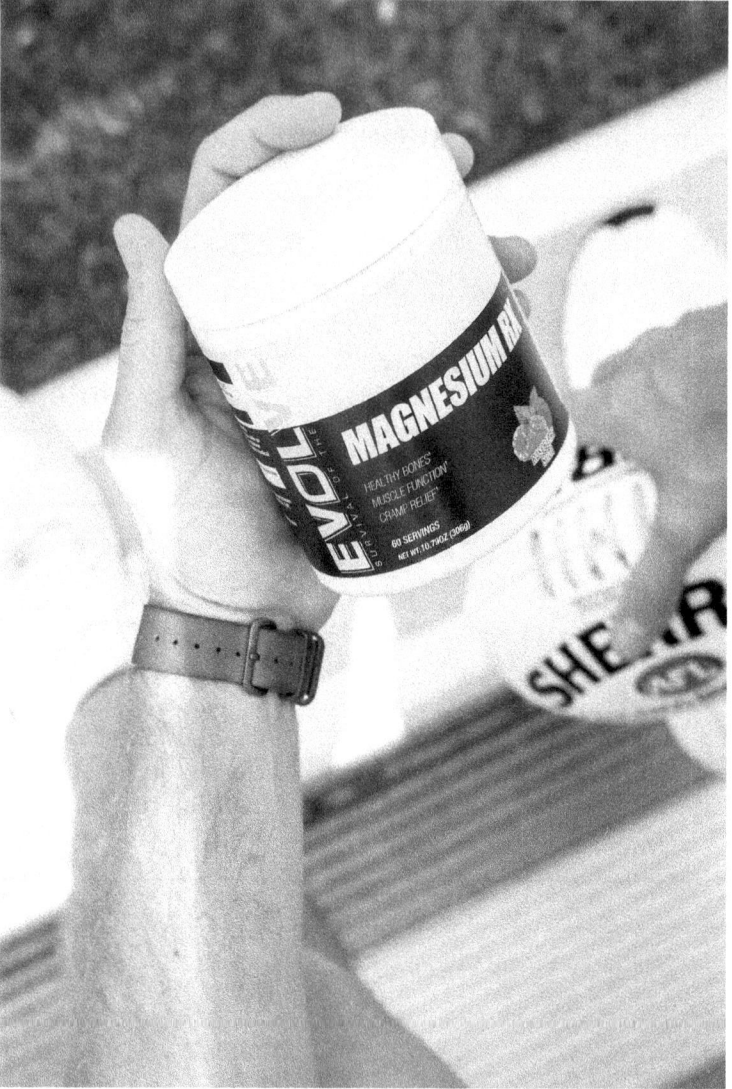

Chapter 7

Medications and Supplements

Common Medications That Affect Heart Rhythm

Common medications can significantly influence heart rhythm, and understanding their effects is crucial for anyone looking to reduce their risk of arrhythmia. Several classes of drugs are known to affect the electrical conduction system of the heart, leading to potential rhythm disturbances. T

hese medications can range from those prescribed for hypertension to over-the-counter remedies that may seem harmless. Being aware of these medications can empower individuals to engage in informed discussions with their healthcare providers.

Beta-blockers are one of the most commonly prescribed medications for managing conditions like hypertension and heart disease. They work by blocking the effects of adrenaline on the heart, which can slow down the heart rate and decrease the heart's workload.

While beneficial for many, beta-blockers can sometimes lead to bradycardia, a condition characterized by an abnormally slow heart rate. Individuals using these medications should monitor their heart rate and report any symptoms of dizziness or fatigue to their healthcare provider.

Antiarrhythmic drugs are specifically designed to treat arrhythmias by stabilizing the electrical activity of the heart. However, they can also have side effects that may complicate heart rhythm. Medications such as amiodarone and sotalol can be effective in controlling certain types of arrhythmias but may also lead to other rhythm disturbances or exacerbate pre-existing conditions. It is essential for patients on these medications to undergo regular follow-up and monitoring to ensure that their heart rhythm remains stable.

Certain antidepressants and antipsychotics have also been linked to changes in heart rhythm. Drugs like selective serotonin reuptake inhibitors (SSRIs) and certain atypical antipsychotics can prolong the QT interval, a specific measure of heart rhythm that, when extended, can lead to serious arrhythmias. Patients should discuss their mental health medications with their healthcare providers, particularly if they have a history of heart disease or arrhythmias, to weigh the benefits against potential risks.

Lastly, over-the-counter medications, including decongestants and some herbal supplements, can also impact heart rhythm. Decongestants like pseudoephedrine can increase heart rate and blood pressure, potentially leading to arrhythmias, especially in sensitive individuals. Likewise, some herbal supplements may interact with prescription medications or have direct effects on heart rhythm.

It is vital for individuals to conduct thorough research and consult healthcare professionals before starting any new medication or supplement, ensuring a comprehensive approach to heart health and arrhythmia prevention.

Heart-Healthy Supplements

Heart-healthy supplements can play a significant role in reducing the risk of arrhythmia. While a balanced diet rich in whole foods is foundational for heart health, certain supplements may offer additional benefits. Omega-3 fatty acids, found in fish oil, are known for their anti-inflammatory properties and ability to lower blood pressure and triglyceride levels.

These fatty acids can help maintain a regular heartbeat and may reduce the frequency of arrhythmias. Individuals considering these supplements should consult with a healthcare provider to determine appropriate dosages and forms that best suit their needs.

Coenzyme Q10 (CoQ10) is another supplement that has garnered attention for its potential cardiovascular benefits. It plays a crucial role in energy production within cells and acts as a powerful antioxidant. Some studies suggest that CoQ10 may help improve heart function, particularly in individuals with heart disease, and can enhance the efficacy of other heart medications.

Regular intake of CoQ10 may help manage the risk factors associated with arrhythmia, such as hypertension and heart failure.

Magnesium is essential for maintaining normal heart rhythm and is often under-consumed in many diets. Supplementation can provide significant benefits, especially for individuals who have low dietary intake or specific health conditions that increase magnesium depletion.

Research indicates that magnesium can help prevent arrhythmias by promoting proper electrical conduction in the heart. As with other supplements, it's important to discuss magnesium supplementation with a healthcare professional, especially for those who have kidney issues or are on medications that may interact with magnesium.

Potassium is another key mineral that supports heart health and rhythm regulation. It helps maintain fluid balance and is critical for muscle contractions, including those of the heart. Adequate potassium levels can help prevent arrhythmias by ensuring that the heart's electrical signals are transmitted effectively.

While potassium can be obtained through dietary sources such as fruits and vegetables, some individuals may benefit from potassium supplements, particularly if they have been diagnosed with deficiencies or are on medications that deplete potassium levels.

Lastly, vitamin D is gaining recognition for its broader implications in cardiovascular health. Emerging research suggests that adequate levels of vitamin D may help reduce the risk of arrhythmias and other heart-related conditions. It is crucial to maintain optimal vitamin D levels, especially for individuals living in areas with limited sunlight exposure.

Regular testing and supplementation, if necessary, can contribute to overall heart health and potentially reduce arrhythmia risk. As always, consultation with a healthcare provider is essential before starting any new supplement regimen.

Consultation with Healthcare Providers

Consultation with healthcare providers is a crucial step in reducing the risk of arrhythmia and maintaining heart health. Engaging with a medical professional allows individuals to gain personalized insights based on their unique health profiles. During these consultations, patients can discuss their medical history, family history of heart conditions, and any symptoms they may be experiencing.

This thorough examination helps in identifying potential risk factors specific to each person, enabling healthcare providers to offer tailored recommendations that can significantly lower the risk of arrhythmias.

In addition to discussing medical history, patients should be prepared to provide details about their lifestyle habits. Factors such as diet, exercise, smoking, and alcohol consumption play a significant role in heart health. Healthcare providers can evaluate these habits and suggest modifications that align with best practices for heart health.

For instance, a diet rich in fruits, vegetables, whole grains, and healthy fats can enhance cardiovascular health and reduce arrhythmia risk. Likewise, incorporating regular physical activity can strengthen the heart and improve overall well-being.

Another essential aspect of these consultations is the potential need for diagnostic testing. Healthcare providers may recommend tests such as an electrocardiogram (ECG), echocardiogram, or Holter monitor to assess heart function and detect any irregularities. These tests provide valuable data that help in developing a comprehensive risk assessment. Understanding the underlying causes of any detected arrhythmias can lead to more effective treatment options and prevention strategies tailored specifically to the individual's needs.

Patients should also engage in open dialogue regarding any medications they are currently taking or considering. Certain medications can influence heart rhythm and may increase the risk of arrhythmia. It is essential for individuals to discuss their complete medication list with their healthcare provider to ensure there are no contraindications or potential side effects that could impact heart health.

Additionally, healthcare providers can offer guidance on the safe use of supplements or alternative therapies that might support heart health without introducing additional risks.

Finally, establishing an ongoing relationship with healthcare providers is vital for continuous monitoring and support. Regular follow-up appointments allow for adjustments in treatment plans as needed and ensure that risk factors are managed effectively over time. Individuals should feel empowered to reach out to their healthcare providers with any concerns or changes in their health status. By fostering this collaborative relationship, patients can stay informed about the best practices for reducing their risk of arrhythmia and achieve better health outcomes.

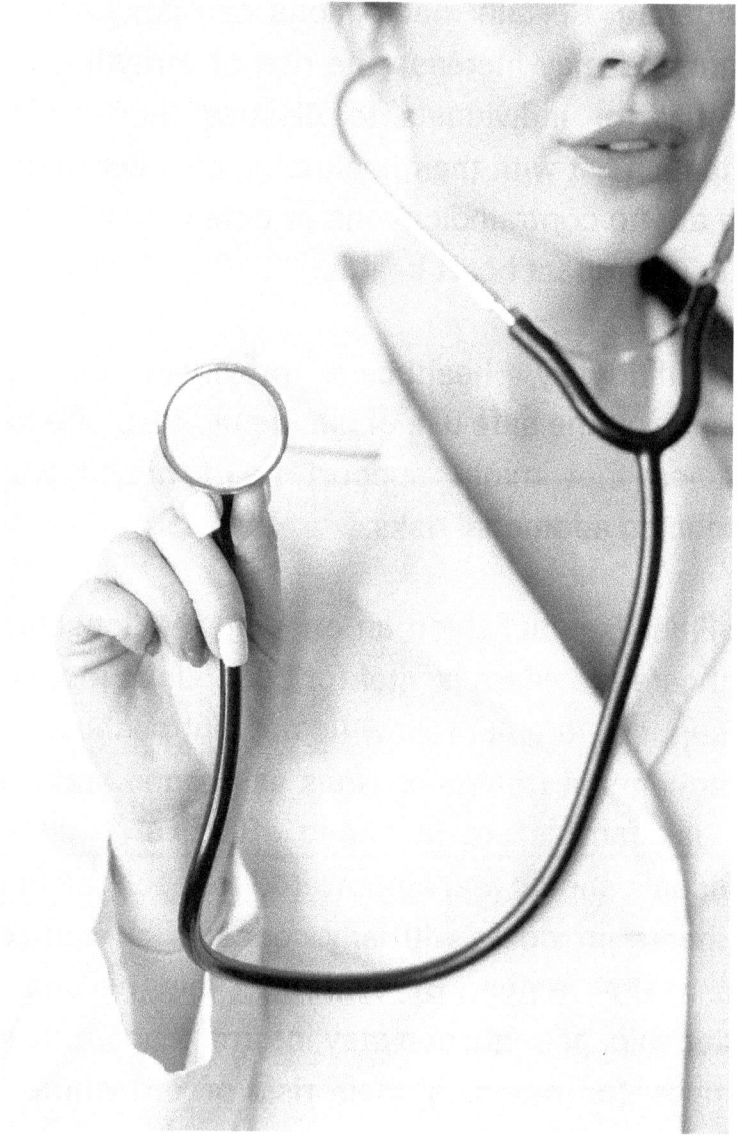

Chapter 8

Monitoring Your Heart Health

Importance of Regular Check-Ups

Regular check-ups play a crucial role in maintaining heart health and reducing the risk of arrhythmia. These routine visits to healthcare providers allow for early detection of potential heart issues before they progress into more serious conditions. During check-ups, healthcare professionals can assess risk factors such as blood pressure, cholesterol levels, and overall cardiovascular health.

Identifying these risks early enables individuals to implement lifestyle changes or medical interventions that can significantly decrease the likelihood of developing arrhythmias.

One of the key benefits of regular check-ups is the opportunity for personalized health assessments. Each person's risk for arrhythmia can vary based on factors such as age, family history, and existing health conditions. Through thorough evaluations, healthcare providers can tailor preventive strategies that align with individual health profiles.

This personalized approach ensures that patients receive the most effective advice and interventions, whether that involves dietary recommendations, exercise plans, or medication management.

Moreover, regular check-ups foster a proactive mindset towards health, encouraging individuals to prioritize their well-being. Knowing that a healthcare professional is monitoring heart health can motivate patients to adhere to healthy lifestyles, including regular exercise and balanced diets. This proactive approach can lead to improved compliance with treatment plans and a greater commitment to heart health, ultimately reducing the risk of arrhythmia and other cardiovascular diseases.

In addition to preventive measures, regular check-ups provide an avenue for education and awareness regarding arrhythmia. Healthcare providers can explain the signs and symptoms of arrhythmias, empowering patients to recognize potential issues early. This knowledge is vital, as timely intervention can prevent complications associated with arrhythmias, such as stroke or heart failure. By understanding their heart health better, individuals are more likely to seek help when necessary.

Lastly, regular check-ups can enhance the doctor-patient relationship, fostering open communication about heart health concerns. This relationship is essential for discussing any symptoms or changes in health, which can significantly impact treatment outcomes.

Patients who feel comfortable discussing their health are more likely to engage actively in their care, leading to better management of risk factors associated with arrhythmia. In summary, regular check-ups are integral to reducing the risk of arrhythmia, promoting health education, and encouraging proactive management of heart health.

Home Monitoring Devices

Home monitoring devices are becoming increasingly popular as essential tools for individuals seeking to manage their heart health and reduce the risk of arrhythmia. These devices enable users to track vital signs and other health metrics from the comfort of their homes.

By offering real-time data on heart rate, blood pressure, and even electrocardiogram (ECG) readings, these gadgets empower users to take proactive steps toward maintaining a healthy heart. Understanding how to effectively utilize these tools can significantly contribute to a comprehensive heart health strategy.

One of the most common home monitoring devices is the heart rate monitor. These devices can be worn as watches or chest straps, providing continuous feedback on heart rate during various activities. Monitoring heart rate is crucial because fluctuations can indicate potential arrhythmias or other cardiovascular issues.

Users can track their resting heart rate, which is a strong indicator of overall heart health. A consistently high resting heart rate may suggest stress, overtraining, or underlying health problems, prompting individuals to consult with healthcare professionals for further evaluation.

Blood pressure monitors are another vital component of home health monitoring. High blood pressure, or hypertension, is a significant risk factor for arrhythmias and other heart conditions. Regularly measuring blood pressure at home allows individuals to identify trends over time, assess the effectiveness of lifestyle changes or medications, and engage in discussions with healthcare providers about their heart health.

Many modern blood pressure monitors offer user-friendly interfaces and can store multiple readings, making it easier to track progress and stay informed about one's cardiovascular status.

Electrocardiogram (ECG) devices have also gained popularity among home health monitoring options. These devices can provide insights into heart rhythm and detect irregularities that may indicate arrhythmia. Some advanced models allow users to take an ECG at home, capturing data that can be shared with healthcare professionals for interpretation.

This capability can be particularly beneficial for individuals who have experienced symptoms of arrhythmia, as it provides objective data that can assist in diagnosis and treatment planning. Understanding one's heart rhythm is crucial for effective management and prevention of arrhythmias.

While home monitoring devices are powerful tools, it is essential to use them correctly and in conjunction with professional medical advice. Individuals should familiarize themselves with the features and limitations of their devices, ensuring that they interpret the data accurately.

Additionally, maintaining open communication with healthcare providers about the readings and any concerning symptoms is vital. This collaborative approach can lead to timely interventions, lifestyle adjustments, or medication changes, all of which are critical for reducing the risk of arrhythmia and promoting overall heart health.

Recognizing Warning Signs

Recognizing warning signs is a crucial step in managing heart health and reducing the risk of arrhythmia. Understanding these signs can empower individuals to seek timely medical attention and implement preventive measures. Early recognition of symptoms can lead to prompt interventions, which may mitigate the progression of heart conditions and enhance overall well-being. Individuals should be familiar with the common warning signs that indicate potential heart rhythm disturbances.

One of the most prevalent warning signs that could point to arrhythmia is palpitations. Palpitations are characterized by a sensation of an irregular heartbeat, which may feel like fluttering, pounding, or racing.

While occasional palpitations can be normal, particularly under stress or excitement, frequent occurrences or those accompanied by dizziness, shortness of breath, or chest pain should prompt a consultation with a healthcare professional. It is essential to differentiate between benign palpitations and those that may signify an underlying issue, as this distinction can influence treatment decisions.

Another significant sign to recognize is fatigue or weakness, particularly if it occurs suddenly or is disproportionate to recent activity levels. This feeling may arise from the heart not pumping effectively, leading to insufficient blood flow to vital organs. Individuals experiencing unexplained fatigue, especially in conjunction with other symptoms like lightheadedness or fainting, should seek medical evaluation.

Understanding that fatigue can be a symptom of arrhythmia can motivate individuals to monitor their health more closely and advocate for necessary assessments.

Chest discomfort is another critical warning sign that should never be ignored. This discomfort may present as tightness, pressure, or a feeling of fullness in the chest and can be associated with arrhythmias. While it is often linked to coronary artery disease, it can also be indicative of various heart rhythm problems.

Individuals should be vigilant about any new or worsening chest pain, particularly if it radiates to the arms, back, neck, or jaw. Recognizing this symptom as a potential warning sign can facilitate timely medical intervention and improve outcomes.

Lastly, it is essential to consider the context of these symptoms in relation to other risk factors. A family history of heart disease, existing health conditions such as high blood pressure or diabetes, and lifestyle factors like smoking or excessive alcohol consumption can exacerbate the risk of arrhythmia. Individuals should be proactive in monitoring their health and recognizing how these risk factors interact with the warning signs. By being informed and alert, individuals can take significant steps toward reducing their risk of arrhythmia and fostering a healthier heart.

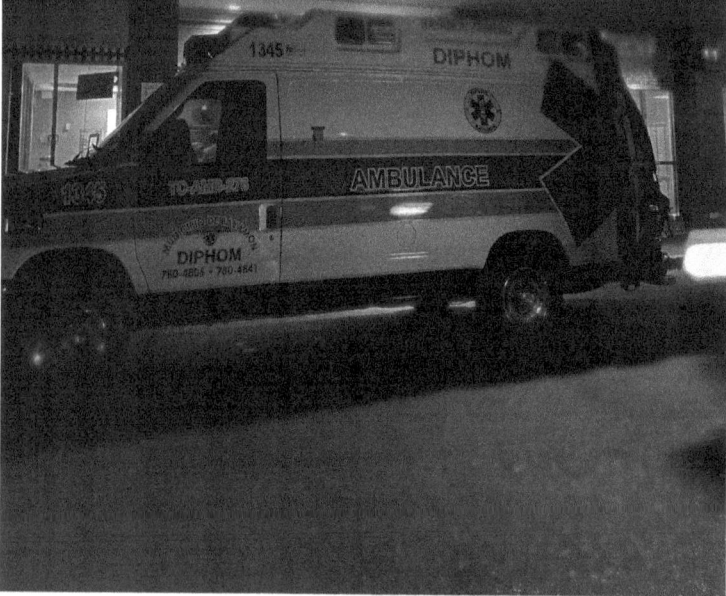

Chapter 9

When to Seek Medical Attention

Understanding Emergency Symptoms

Understanding the symptoms of an emergency related to arrhythmias is crucial for anyone looking to reduce their risk of heart complications. Arrhythmias, or irregular heartbeats, can manifest in various ways, and recognizing these symptoms can be life-saving. The heart may beat too quickly, too slowly, or in an irregular pattern, and each of these scenarios can signal a potential emergency.

It is important for individuals to familiarize themselves with what constitutes an emergency symptom versus a benign condition.

Common emergency symptoms associated with arrhythmias include chest pain, shortness of breath, dizziness, and fainting. Chest pain, often described as pressure or a squeezing sensation, can indicate that the heart is not receiving enough oxygen. Shortness of breath can occur suddenly and may be accompanied by a feeling of tightness in the chest.

Dizziness or lightheadedness may occur due to inadequate blood flow to the brain, potentially leading to fainting. Recognizing these signs early can prompt timely medical intervention, which is essential for improving outcomes.

In addition to the more obvious symptoms, there are also less common signs that may indicate an urgent situation. Palpitations, or the feeling of a racing heart, can be alarming, especially when accompanied by other symptoms, such as anxiety or sweating. Some individuals may experience extreme fatigue or weakness, which can be misleading as these symptoms might be attributed to other causes.

It is vital to note these feelings and seek help if they persist or worsen. Understanding the full spectrum of symptoms can empower individuals to respond appropriately.

It is also important to understand that not all symptoms signify a life-threatening condition, but they should never be ignored. Some people may experience irregular heartbeats without any severe symptoms and may not require immediate medical attention.

However, if these irregularities are new or have changed in intensity or frequency, it is advisable to consult a healthcare professional. Continuous monitoring of one's heart health and being aware of personal symptoms can lead to better management and prevention strategies.

Education on emergency symptoms can significantly enhance one's ability to act swiftly in critical situations. Individuals should consider keeping a symptom diary to track any irregularities in heart rhythm, how they feel during these episodes, and any related activities or stressors.

This record can be invaluable during consultations with healthcare providers, allowing for a better understanding of one's heart health and potentially leading to preventive measures tailored to individual needs. By being proactive in recognizing and understanding emergency symptoms, individuals can take significant steps toward reducing their risk of arrhythmia and enhancing their overall heart health.

Preparing for Doctor Visits

Preparing for a doctor visit is a crucial step in managing your heart health and reducing the risk of arrhythmia. Before your appointment, it's essential to compile a comprehensive list of your symptoms, medical history, and any medications you are currently taking.

This preparation not only saves time but also ensures that your healthcare provider has all the necessary information to make an informed diagnosis. Symptoms such as palpitations, dizziness, or fatigue should be noted, along with their frequency and duration, to provide insight into your heart health.

In addition to listing symptoms, it is important to bring along your medical history. This includes previous diagnoses, surgeries, and family history of heart conditions. Understanding your family's health history can be vital, as certain types of arrhythmias can have a genetic component.

If you have had any previous tests related to your heart health, such as an electrocardiogram (ECG) or echocardiogram, be sure to request copies of these results to share with your doctor.

Another key aspect of preparation is to write down any questions or concerns you may have. This can range from inquiries about lifestyle changes, dietary recommendations, or the need for further testing. Having specific questions prepared allows you to maximize your time with the doctor and ensures that you leave the appointment with a clear understanding of your heart health.

It can also be beneficial to bring a family member or friend to the appointment, as they can provide support and help remember the information discussed.

Prior to your visit, consider keeping a diary of your daily activities, diet, and any occurrences of symptoms. This log can provide valuable context for your doctor regarding how your lifestyle may be impacting your heart health. By tracking your physical activity, stress levels, and sleep patterns, you may identify potential triggers for any arrhythmia symptoms you experience. This information can lead to more tailored recommendations from your healthcare provider.

Finally, be open and honest during your appointment. Your doctor is there to help you, and providing truthful information about your lifestyle choices, habits, and concerns will allow them to offer the best possible guidance. Discussing any fears or misconceptions you may have about your heart health can also foster a more productive dialogue.

By being proactive in your preparation for doctor visits, you empower yourself to take control of your health and actively work towards reducing your risk of arrhythmia.

Treatment Options for Arrhythmia

Treatment options for arrhythmia vary widely, depending on the type and severity of the condition. For those seeking to reduce their risk of arrhythmia, understanding these options is crucial. The first line of defense often includes lifestyle modifications.

Maintaining a heart-healthy diet rich in fruits, vegetables, whole grains, and lean proteins can help regulate heart rhythm. Regular physical activity, such as walking or cycling, can improve cardiovascular health and reduce stress, both of which are vital in minimizing arrhythmic episodes.

In addition to lifestyle changes, medications play a significant role in the management of arrhythmias. Antiarrhythmic drugs are commonly prescribed to restore the heart's normal rhythm or to control heart rate. These medications work by altering the electrical signals in the heart and may include beta-blockers, calcium channel blockers, and sodium channel blockers.

It's essential for patients to work closely with their healthcare providers to find the most effective medication with the fewest side effects, as individual responses to these drugs can vary.

For those who do not respond adequately to medication, more invasive procedures may be necessary. Catheter ablation is a minimally invasive procedure that involves threading a catheter through the blood vessels to the heart. This technique aims to destroy small areas of heart tissue that are causing abnormal electrical signals.

For some patients, this can provide a long-term solution to recurrent arrhythmias. Another option is the implantation of a pacemaker, a device that helps regulate the heart's rhythm by sending electrical impulses to the heart as needed.

In severe cases of arrhythmia, especially those that lead to life-threatening conditions, surgical interventions may be considered. Surgical options include the maze procedure, where a surgeon creates scar tissue in the heart to disrupt abnormal electrical pathways, or the installation of an implantable cardioverter-defibrillator (ICD). An ICD monitors the heart's rhythm and delivers shocks when it detects dangerous arrhythmias, effectively preventing sudden cardiac arrest.

Emphasizing prevention through education and awareness is crucial for individuals looking to minimize their risk of arrhythmia. Regular check-ups with a healthcare provider can help identify potential risk factors early, allowing for timely intervention.

By understanding the various treatment options available, individuals can collaborate with their healthcare team to establish a comprehensive plan tailored to their specific needs and risks, ultimately fostering a healthier heart.

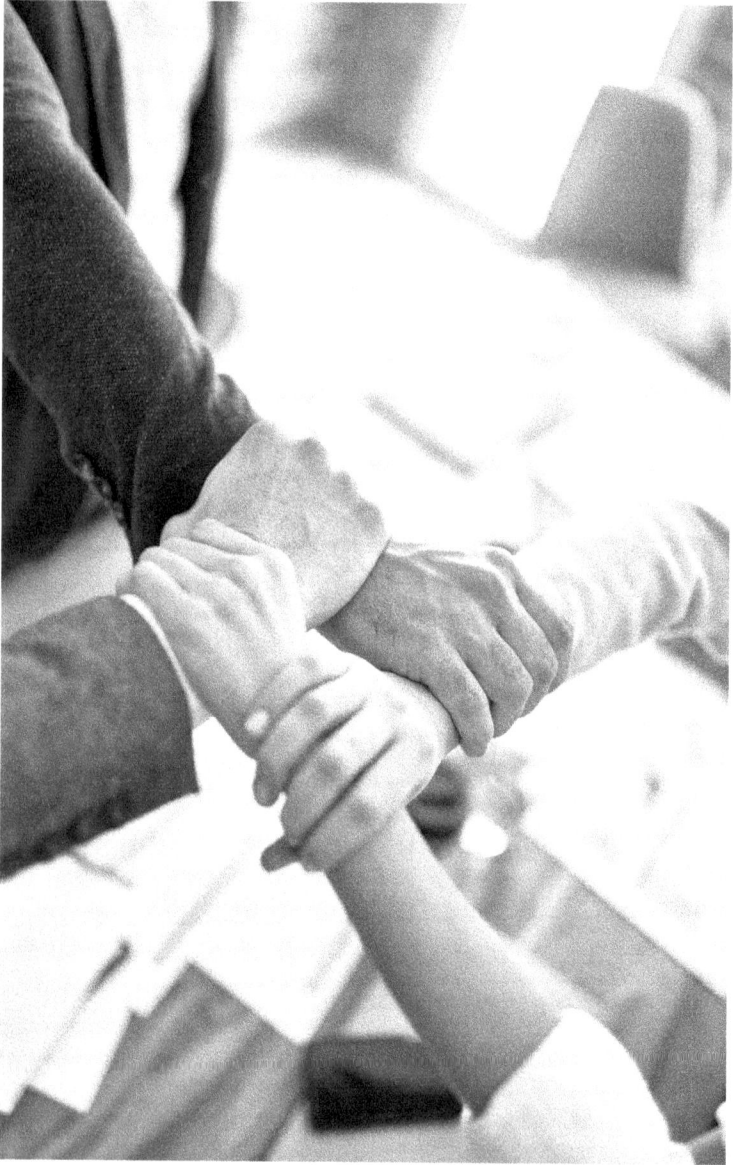

Chapter 10

Building a Support System

The Role of Family and Friends

The support of family and friends plays a crucial role in reducing the risk of arrhythmia. Emotional and practical assistance from loved ones can significantly enhance an individual's ability to make heart-healthy choices. When family and friends are actively engaged in promoting heart health, they can help create an environment that encourages positive lifestyle changes.

This supportive network can provide motivation and accountability, making it easier for individuals to adhere to recommended dietary and exercise regimens that contribute to cardiovascular health.

Healthy communication within families and among friends is vital in promoting awareness about arrhythmia and its risk factors. By sharing knowledge about heart health, individuals can better understand the importance of maintaining a healthy lifestyle. Conversations can also facilitate discussions about medical history, including any hereditary conditions that may increase the risk of arrhythmia.

This awareness allows individuals to take proactive steps in managing their health, such as scheduling regular check-ups and discussing any concerns with healthcare providers.

Family and friends can also play a pivotal role in encouraging participation in heart-healthy activities. Engaging in physical exercise together, such as walking, cycling, or joining fitness classes, not only improves cardiovascular fitness but also strengthens social bonds.

These shared experiences can make exercising more enjoyable and less daunting, thereby increasing adherence to regular physical activity.

Additionally, cooking healthy meals together can foster better eating habits and provide opportunities for learning about nutrition, ultimately contributing to heart health.

In times of stress, which can be a trigger for arrhythmia, having a strong support system becomes even more critical. Family and friends can help individuals navigate stressful situations by providing emotional support and practical strategies for stress management. Techniques such as mindfulness, meditation, or simply having someone to talk to can mitigate stress levels. Encouraging loved ones to participate in relaxation activities together can further enhance resilience against the physiological effects of stress on the heart.

Lastly, the role of family and friends extends to providing ongoing encouragement and reinforcement of heart-healthy habits. Celebrating small victories in lifestyle changes helps individuals stay motivated on their journey toward a healthier heart.

Whether it is acknowledging weight loss achievements, improvements in fitness levels, or maintaining a balanced diet, these positive reinforcements can build confidence and a sense of accomplishment. By fostering a culture of health and well-being within their social circles, individuals are more likely to sustain the lifestyle changes necessary to reduce their risk of arrhythmia.

Support Groups and Resources

Support groups and resources play a crucial role in managing heart health, particularly for individuals looking to reduce their risk of arrhythmia. These platforms provide not only emotional support but also practical information and shared experiences that can empower individuals on their journey towards a healthier heart.

Many people find comfort and motivation in connecting with others who face similar challenges, which can facilitate a positive change in lifestyle and attitudes towards heart health.

One of the most effective ways to find support is through local or online support groups specifically geared towards heart health or arrhythmia management. These groups often include members who have experienced arrhythmia or other heart-related conditions, and they foster a sense of community.

Participants can share their stories, discuss coping strategies, and exchange information about what has worked for them. In addition to emotional support, these groups frequently invite healthcare professionals to provide insights, answer questions, and suggest lifestyle modifications that can help mitigate risks associated with arrhythmia.

Several national and local organizations offer resources for those at risk of arrhythmia. These organizations typically provide educational materials, workshops, and seminars focused on heart health. They may also facilitate access to webinars featuring medical professionals who specialize in cardiology.

These resources not only enhance knowledge about arrhythmia and its risk factors but also promote awareness of the latest research and treatment options available. Engaging with these organizations can help individuals stay informed and motivated to implement preventative strategies in their daily lives.

In addition to support groups and organizations, online resources and forums can be invaluable for those seeking to reduce their risk of arrhythmia. Websites dedicated to heart health often feature articles, videos, and interactive tools that help users understand their heart health better.

Many forums allow individuals to connect with others globally, offering a broader perspective on living with arrhythmia or managing heart health. These digital platforms can be particularly beneficial for those who may have difficulty accessing in-person resources or who prefer the convenience of online engagement.

Lastly, it is essential to recognize the importance of professional guidance when exploring support groups and resources. Consulting with healthcare providers can ensure that individuals choose the right groups or organizations that align with their specific needs. Physicians can recommend reputable sources and may even facilitate introductions to local support groups.

By combining the advantages of community support with expert advice, individuals can create a comprehensive approach to reducing their risk of arrhythmia, ultimately leading to improved heart health and overall well-being.

Mental Health Support

Mental health plays a crucial role in maintaining overall heart health, including reducing the risk of arrhythmia. Stress, anxiety, and depression can significantly impact heart health, leading to increased heart rate and other physiological changes that may contribute to arrhythmias.

Understanding the connection between mental health and heart health is essential for individuals looking to minimize their risk of developing heart rhythm disorders. By addressing mental health proactively, individuals can enhance their emotional well-being and contribute to better cardiovascular outcomes.

One effective strategy for supporting mental health is mindfulness and stress reduction techniques. Practices such as meditation, yoga, and deep-breathing exercises can help lower stress levels, promote relaxation, and improve emotional stability.

These techniques not only reduce anxiety but also positively influence heart rate variability, a key factor in maintaining a healthy heart rhythm. Regularly incorporating mindfulness practices into daily routines can create a buffer against stress, which is particularly beneficial for those at risk of arrhythmia.

Social support also plays a vital role in mental health. Connecting with friends, family, and support groups can provide emotional reassurance and decrease feelings of isolation, which can exacerbate stress and anxiety.

Engaging in social activities and maintaining strong relationships can foster a sense of belonging and security. For individuals concerned about arrhythmia, discussing their fears and experiences with loved ones can alleviate anxiety and promote a more positive outlook on their health.

Professional mental health support, such as therapy or counseling, can be invaluable for those struggling with significant stress, anxiety, or depression. Mental health professionals can offer tailored strategies to manage emotions and develop coping skills.

Cognitive-behavioral therapy (CBT), for instance, has been shown to be effective in reducing anxiety and improving overall mental well-being. By addressing mental health concerns with professional guidance, individuals can better equip themselves to face the challenges associated with arrhythmia risk.

Finally, lifestyle modifications that support both mental and physical health are essential for reducing the risk of arrhythmia.

Regular physical activity, a balanced diet, adequate sleep, and avoiding harmful substances such as tobacco and excessive alcohol can significantly improve mental health. These lifestyle changes not only enhance mood and reduce stress but also contribute to cardiovascular health, creating a comprehensive approach to minimizing arrhythmia risk. By prioritizing mental wellness as part of a holistic heart health strategy, individuals can foster resilience and empower themselves on their journey toward a healthier heart.

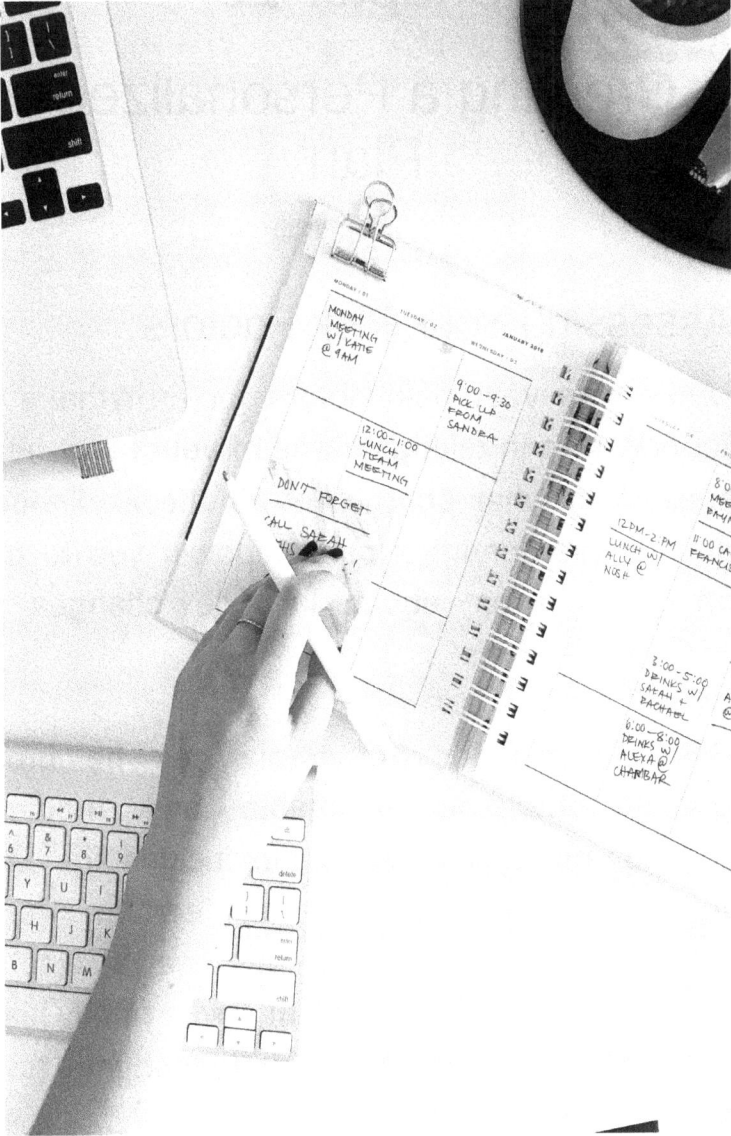

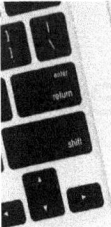

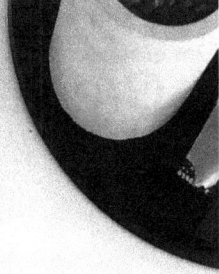

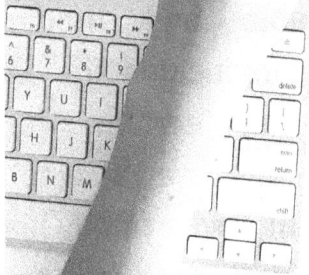

Chapter 11

Creating a Personalized Plan

Assessing Your Risk Factors

Assessing your risk factors for arrhythmia is a crucial first step in taking charge of your heart health. Understanding what contributes to the likelihood of developing this condition can empower you to make informed decisions about lifestyle changes and medical interventions.

Risk factors for arrhythmia can be broadly categorized into non-modifiable and modifiable factors. Non-modifiable risk factors include age, family history of heart disease, and certain genetic predispositions. As you age, the heart's electrical system may become less efficient, and a family history of arrhythmias can indicate a genetic tendency toward heart rhythm disturbances.

Modifiable risk factors, on the other hand, are those that you can influence through lifestyle choices and medical management. Common modifiable risk factors include hypertension, smoking, obesity, excessive alcohol consumption, and sedentary behavior. Managing blood pressure through diet, exercise, and medication can significantly reduce your risk.

Additionally, quitting smoking, maintaining a healthy weight, and limiting alcohol intake are all actionable steps that can lower your chances of developing arrhythmias. Evaluating your lifestyle habits is essential, as these choices play a critical role in heart health.

Another aspect of assessing your risk involves monitoring existing health conditions. Conditions such as diabetes, thyroid disorders, and sleep apnea can increase the likelihood of arrhythmias. Regular check-ups with your healthcare provider can help identify these conditions early and allow for timely intervention.

If you have already been diagnosed with such conditions, working closely with your healthcare team to manage them effectively is vital. This proactive approach can help mitigate your risk and promote overall cardiovascular health.

Stress management is also an important factor in assessing your risk for arrhythmia. Chronic stress can impact heart health by increasing blood pressure and heart rate, which may contribute to irregular heart rhythms.

Implementing stress-reducing techniques such as mindfulness, meditation, and regular physical activity can be beneficial. It is essential to recognize the signs of stress and take steps to manage it effectively as part of your overall risk assessment and reduction strategy.

Finally, it is important to engage in regular heart health screenings and discuss your risk factors with your healthcare provider. They can provide personalized recommendations based on your individual risk profile.

Keeping track of your heart health through regular monitoring and open communication with your medical team can help you stay informed about your risk factors and make necessary adjustments. By taking these steps, you can significantly reduce your risk of arrhythmia and work towards a healthier heart.

Setting Goals for a Healthier Heart

Setting goals for a healthier heart is a crucial step in reducing the risk of arrhythmia. When individuals take the time to identify and establish specific, measurable, achievable, relevant, and time-bound (SMART) goals, they create a structured approach to improving their cardiovascular health.

This method not only enhances motivation but also provides a clear roadmap for making sustainable lifestyle changes. By focusing on heart health, individuals can significantly lower their chances of developing arrhythmias and other heart-related issues.

One of the first steps in setting effective goals is to assess current health status. Understanding baseline metrics such as blood pressure, cholesterol levels, and body weight can help individuals identify areas for improvement. For example, if an individual discovers they have high cholesterol, a relevant goal might be to lower it by a specific percentage over a defined period. Regular check-ups and consultations with healthcare providers can help monitor progress and adjust goals as necessary, ensuring that they remain realistic and attainable.

Incorporating physical activity into daily routines is another vital goal for heart health. The American Heart Association recommends at least 150 minutes of moderate aerobic exercise per week. Setting a goal to engage in physical activity for a certain number of days each week can be a great way to stay accountable.

This could include activities such as walking, cycling, swimming, or any other form of exercise that raises the heart rate. Individuals should aim to find activities they enjoy, as this increases the likelihood of maintaining consistency and making exercise a lifelong habit.

Dietary changes are equally important in achieving heart health goals. Setting specific targets, such as increasing the intake of fruits and vegetables or reducing sodium consumption, can lead to significant improvements in cardiovascular health. Individuals might choose to set a goal to prepare homemade meals a certain number of times each week, focusing on whole, unprocessed foods.

Educating oneself about nutrition and understanding how different foods affect heart health can further empower individuals to make informed choices that align with their goals.

Finally, managing stress and prioritizing mental well-being play significant roles in heart health. Goals in this area might include practicing mindfulness, engaging in regular relaxation techniques, or dedicating time to hobbies that bring joy. Establishing routines that incorporate stress-reducing activities can help mitigate the impact of stress on the heart. By recognizing the interconnectedness of physical and mental health, individuals can foster a holistic approach to reducing their risk of arrhythmia, ultimately leading to a healthier heart and improved overall well-being.

Regularly Updating Your Plan

Regularly updating your plan is a crucial component in the journey to reduce the risk of arrhythmia. As new research emerges and guidelines evolve, it is essential to stay informed about the latest findings related to heart health.

A well-informed approach allows individuals to make necessary adjustments in their lifestyle, medication, and overall health strategies. By keeping abreast of advancements in medical science, you can ensure your plan remains effective and aligned with current best practices.

Monitoring your health metrics is an important aspect of this process. Regular check-ups with your healthcare provider can offer insights into your heart health and help identify any changes that may require adjustments to your plan. For example, fluctuations in blood pressure, cholesterol levels, or weight can all influence your risk of arrhythmia. Maintaining an open dialogue with your healthcare team will enable you to tailor your strategies based on your unique health profile and any emerging health conditions.

In addition to medical evaluations, consider personal reflections and lifestyle assessments as part of your plan updates. Regularly reviewing your dietary habits, exercise routines, and stress management techniques will help you identify areas that may need improvement.

Establishing a habit of self-reflection can also empower you to recognize triggers that may lead to arrhythmia, allowing you to proactively address them. Journaling your experiences can be a useful tool to track your progress and pinpoint behaviors that need modification.

Furthermore, staying connected with support networks can enrich your knowledge and motivate you to keep your plan current. Engaging with community groups, online forums, or patient education programs can provide you with up-to-date information and shared experiences from others who are also working to reduce their risk of arrhythmia. These interactions can foster a sense of accountability and encourage you to remain committed to your health goals, ensuring that your strategies evolve along with your understanding of heart health.

Lastly, consider incorporating technology into your approach. Many apps and digital platforms are designed to help monitor heart health and track lifestyle changes. These tools can facilitate regular updates to your plan by providing real-time data and reminders for healthy behaviors. Leveraging technology not only helps you stay on track but also empowers you to make informed decisions based on your ongoing health journey.

By regularly updating your plan, you can create a dynamic, responsive strategy that adapts to your needs and enhances your overall heart health.

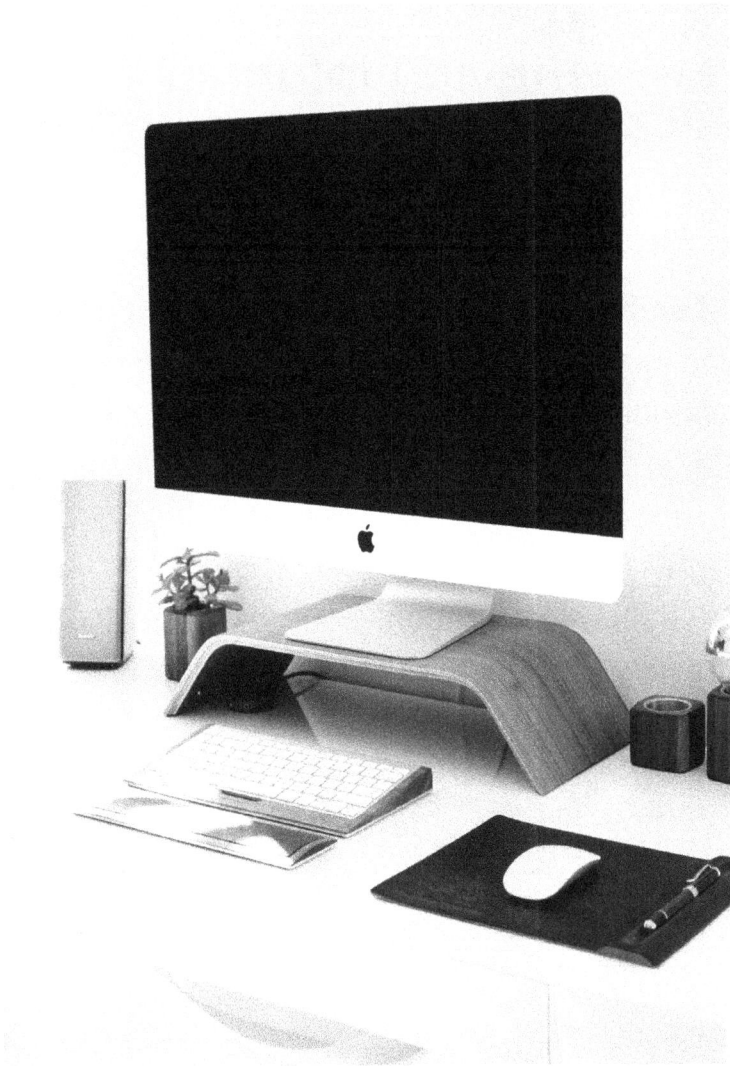

Chapter 12

Staying Informed

Reliable Sources of Information

Reliable sources of information are crucial for anyone looking to reduce their risk of arrhythmia. With the abundance of health information available online and in print, it can be challenging to discern which sources are credible and trustworthy.

Reliable information sources typically include peer-reviewed medical journals, established health organizations, and healthcare professionals. These sources are grounded in research and provide insights that are both evidence-based and up to date, ensuring that readers receive accurate information regarding heart health and arrhythmia prevention.

One of the most authoritative sources for heart health information is the American Heart Association (AHA). The AHA provides extensive resources on cardiovascular health, including guidelines on lifestyle changes that can reduce the risk of arrhythmias. Their publications are widely recognized and are often authored by experts in the field.

By consulting the AHA's materials, individuals can access a wealth of information on dietary recommendations, exercise regimens, and management strategies for existing heart conditions, all of which can contribute to a healthier heart.

In addition to organizations like the AHA, peer-reviewed journals such as the Journal of the American College of Cardiology and Circulation publish the latest research findings related to heart health. These journals are essential for anyone looking to understand the scientific basis behind arrhythmia prevention strategies.

They often include studies that explore the effects of various interventions, ranging from lifestyle modifications to medical treatments, on arrhythmia rates and heart health overall. Staying informed through these publications can help individuals make educated decisions about their health.

Healthcare professionals, including cardiologists and primary care physicians, are invaluable sources of personalized information regarding heart health. Consulting with a healthcare provider allows individuals to discuss their specific risk factors and receive tailored advice.

Doctors can interpret the latest research and apply it to individual circumstances, helping patients understand how to implement changes that will effectively reduce their risk of arrhythmia. Regular consultations with healthcare professionals ensure that individuals remain informed about the latest developments in heart health.

Lastly, reputable health websites can serve as supplementary resources for information on arrhythmia prevention. Websites belonging to established health institutions or government health agencies often provide fact-checked articles, guidelines, and resources that can help individuals navigate their heart health journey. However, it is important to remain cautious and verify the credibility of online sources, as misinformation can easily proliferate on the internet.

By prioritizing reliable sources of information, individuals can empower themselves with the knowledge needed to effectively reduce their risk of arrhythmia and foster long-term heart health.

The Importance of Continuing Education

Continuing education plays a vital role in empowering individuals to take control of their heart health, particularly in the context of reducing the risk of arrhythmia.

As new research emerges and medical guidelines evolve, staying informed about the latest findings and treatment options becomes crucial. Individuals who prioritize learning about heart health can better understand their own risk factors, recognize symptoms, and adopt effective preventive measures. This proactive approach not only enhances personal knowledge but also fosters a sense of agency over one's health journey.

One of the key benefits of continuing education is the ability to access evidence-based information. Many resources, including online courses, workshops, and community health programs, are available to those seeking to deepen their understanding of arrhythmia and related conditions.

By engaging with reputable sources, individuals can learn about the physiological mechanisms behind arrhythmias, the importance of lifestyle factors such as diet and exercise, and the role of stress management in heart health. This comprehensive understanding helps individuals make informed choices that can significantly impact their risk levels.

Moreover, continuing education encourages individuals to stay updated on advancements in treatment and management strategies for arrhythmia. Medical professionals regularly revise their recommendations based on the latest research studies, and being aware of these changes can lead to better health outcomes.

For instance, advancements in technology have introduced new monitoring devices and treatment options that can help manage arrhythmias more effectively. Individuals who actively seek out this knowledge can engage in meaningful conversations with healthcare providers, advocating for the best treatment options tailored to their specific needs.

Participating in educational opportunities can also foster a supportive community among individuals with similar health concerns. Group classes, health seminars, and online forums allow people to share experiences, strategies, and personal stories related to managing arrhythmia.

This sense of community not only provides emotional support but also enhances motivation to maintain heart-healthy habits. When individuals see others making progress in their health journeys, they are often inspired to adopt similar practices, creating a ripple effect that promotes collective well-being.

Finally, the importance of continuing education extends beyond personal benefits; it contributes to broader public health awareness. As more individuals become educated about arrhythmia and its risk factors, there is a greater likelihood of increased advocacy for heart health initiatives within communities.

This collective effort can lead to improved access to resources, better healthcare policies, and enhanced prevention programs that benefit everyone. By prioritizing continuing education, individuals not only enhance their own health but also play a crucial role in fostering a healthier society.

Engaging with Healthcare Professionals

Engaging with healthcare professionals is a crucial step in reducing the risk of arrhythmia. Building a collaborative relationship with your medical team empowers you to take an active role in your heart health. Begin by selecting a healthcare provider who specializes in cardiology or has experience in treating heart rhythm disorders.

Consider their qualifications, experience, and communication style to ensure they align with your needs and preferences. A good rapport with your healthcare provider will encourage open discussions about your health concerns, lifestyle choices, and potential risk factors for arrhythmia.

During your visits, it is important to come prepared with a list of questions and concerns regarding your heart health. This might include inquiries about your family history of heart conditions, symptoms you may be experiencing, or lifestyle changes you are considering.

Taking notes during consultations can help you remember important information and recommendations. Don't hesitate to seek clarification on medical jargon or suggested treatments. A proactive approach not only enhances your understanding but also demonstrates your commitment to managing your heart health effectively.

Regular check-ups and screenings play a vital role in identifying risk factors for arrhythmia early on. Engaging in preventive care allows healthcare professionals to monitor your heart health over time. Discuss with your provider how often you should schedule these visits based on your personal health history and lifestyle.

Ensure that you adhere to any recommended tests, such as an electrocardiogram (ECG) or Holter monitor, which can provide valuable insights into your heart's rhythm and help detect potential issues before they escalate.

Lifestyle modifications are integral to reducing the risk of arrhythmia, and healthcare professionals can guide you in making these changes. Discuss your diet, exercise routine, and stress management techniques with your provider. They can offer tailored advice based on your individual circumstances, helping you develop a sustainable plan to improve your overall heart health. Additionally, they can connect you with nutritionists, physical therapists, or support groups to enhance your efforts in making healthy choices.

Finally, it is essential to stay informed about your condition and treatment options. Engage with your healthcare professionals about the latest research and advancements in arrhythmia management. They can recommend reputable resources, including websites, books, or community programs that can further your understanding.

By fostering an ongoing dialogue with your healthcare team, you not only enhance your knowledge but also empower yourself to make informed decisions that contribute to a healthier heart and a reduced risk of arrhythmia.

Author Notes & Acknowledgments

First and foremost, I would like to express my deepest gratitude to the people who inspired and supported me throughout the journey of writing this book. This project would not have been possible without their unwavering belief in me and their invaluable contributions.

To my wife, thank you for your constant encouragement and understanding. Your love and support have been my anchor during the challenging times of researching and writing this book. Your belief in my ability to make a difference in people's lives has been my driving force.

I would also like to disclose that this book contains some renewed artificial intelligence-generated content. I really appreciate very recent technological innovation by outstanding scientists and of course our reader's understanding.

Lastly, I want to express my deepest gratitude to the readers of this book. I sincerely hope the strategies and methods outlined within these pages will provide you with the knowledge and tools needed to truly make your life much better. Your commitment to seeking any good solutions and willingness to explore multiple methods is commendable.

Author Bio

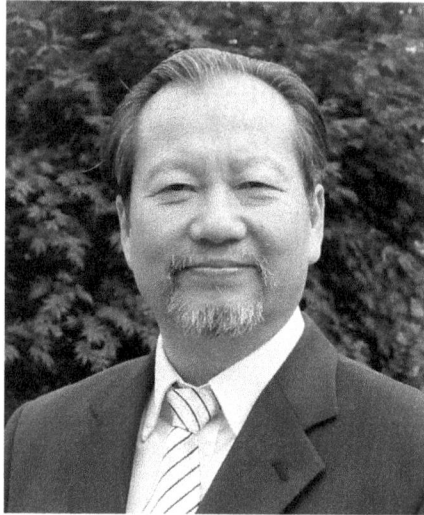

Johnson Wu earned his MD in 1982. With over 40 years of clinical experience, he has worked in hospitals in Zhejiang and Shanghai, China, as well as the Royal Marsden Hospital (part of Imperial College) in London, UK. Upon the recommendation of Sir Aaron Klug, the president of The Royal Society and a Nobel Prize winner in Chemistry, Dr. Wu was honorably awarded a British Royal Society Fellowship. He has published over 100 medical books in many countries and currently practices medicine in Canada.

www.ingramcontent.com/pod-product-compliance
Lightning Source LLC
Chambersburg PA
CBHW060239030426

42335CB00014B/1532